Dance and Stress:

Judith Lynne Hanna (Ph.D., Columbia), a senior research scholar at University of Maryland and a consultant in the arts, education, health, and public policy, practices an anthropology that interrelates multidisciplinary theory, research, and application. Author of *To Dance Is Human* (University of Chicago Press, 1987, reprint of 1979), *The Performer-Audience Connection* (University of Texas Press, 1983), *Disruptive School Behavior* (Holmes & Meier, 1988), *Dance, Sex, and Gender* (University of Chicago Press, 1988), and more than three-score scholarly and other articles, as well as co-author of *Urban Dynamics in Black Africa* (Aldine, 1981), she has taught and lectured at numerous universities in the United States and abroad.

STRESS IN
MODERN SOCIETY
Number 13

Dance and Stress
Resistance, Reduction, and Euphoria

Judith Lynne Hanna

Senior Research Scholar
University of Maryland

AMS PRESS, INC.
New York

Stress in Modern Society: No. 13

Other Titles in This Series:
No. 1. James H. Humphrey, ed. *Stress in Childhood,* 1984.
No. 2. James H. Humphrey, *Profiles in Stress,* 1986.
No. 3. Joy N. Humphrey and James H. Humphrey. *Coping with Stress in Teaching,* 1986.
No. 4. George S. Everly, Jr. and Stephen A. Sobelman. *Assessment of the Human Stress Response,* 1987.
No. 6. Jerrold S. Greenberg. *Stress and Sexuality,* 1987.

Library of Congress Cataloging-in-Publication Data

Hanna, Judith Lynne.
  Dance and stress.

  (Stress in modern society; no. 13)
  Bibliography: p.
  Includes index.
  1. Dancing—Psychology aspects. 2. Stress (Psychology)
3. Dance therapy. I. Title. II. Series.
GV1588.5.H36 1988   793.3'01   86-82028
ISBN 0-404-63264-5

AMS Press, Inc.
56 East 13th Street
New York, N.Y. 10003

MANUFACTURED IN THE UNITED STATES OF AMERICA

Contents

Part II: Illustrative Historical and
Non-Western Dance–Stress Relations

Preface

Hardly a day passes that one is not reminded of stress. We experience it, the news media report it, medical researchers investigate it. Many difficulties previously labelled in various ways are now subsumed under the term *stress*. A fact of modern society with its shattering changes (see Toffler, 1970), stress has been part of human existence from the time of our earliest records. And since early history, dance has been one means to cope with stress. Today dance is among several techniques, such as body movement, role-playing, and relaxation, that people use for this purpose.

Why dance rather than other forms of exercise or passive approaches to handle stress? Dance seems to have special characteristics that I point out in Chapter 1. Indeed, to dance is human. Cave paintings and artifacts with images of dance document its antiquity. Later historical records attest to the persistence of this phenomenon into the contemporary era. Even when dance has been repressed or suppressed, it reappears like a phoenix.

This book will describe some of the palette of dance experience, forms and practices, that individuals and groups through history and around the world have drawn upon to adapt creatively to the exigencies of survival. Chapter 2 describes three key relationships between dance and stress, types of stress management approaches, styles of intervention in stress reactivity, and dance genres associated with stress reactivity. Part II (Chapters 3 to 7), with its presentation of dance practices related to stress that come from cultures different in many ways from our own, can help us better understand ourselves and draw upon what seems to have benefitted others.

Part III turns to contemporary Western society. Chapter 8 focuses on how choreographers, dancers, and audiences manage stress through the medium of theatrical stage performance. Chapter 9 examines stressors in pursuing a professional dance career. Amateur dancers, too, deal with stress, as Chapter 10 illustrates. Dance in its therapeutic manifestations is the subject of Chapter 11. Guidelines for dancing without injury and for managing stress appear in the Conclusion.

The intended audience for this book includes fitness devotees, dancers, health practitioners, scholars and students in the arts, humanities, and social and behavioral sciences, as well as anyone interested in dance or health. Because I have written the book with a broad readership in mind, specialists may find certain sections familiar or even elementary. I beg their patience; the familiar material, I hope, will offer a comfortable map before moving into foreign terrain. As a pioneer study, this work should catalyze further exploration.

A book is the result of an author's exchanges with other people. Among these who have been especially helpful, I wish to thank James H. Humphrey, Diane Dulicai, Brad D. Hatfield, Linda Valleroy, Mary Moore Free, Irini Nadel Rockwell, Lynnette Overby, Carol Martin, Ilene Ava Serlin, Cynthia Novack, Barry Laine, Joan and Barry Stahl, and Jennifer Predock-Linnell for generously sharing resources and observations; the University of Maryland libraries for their multiple services; Judy White for responding to portions of the manuscript, and Predock-Linnell, Overby, Thomas F. Johnston, Luana Kaufmann, and Frances Davidson for their comments on earlier drafts. Much appreciation goes to Serlin, who insightfully critiqued the study from the perspectives of a dance therapist and a psychologist.

The University of Texas Press is gratefully acknowledged for permission to quote short selections from *The Performer-Audience Connection.*

PART I

Setting the Stage

This section explains the purpose of the book, the concepts of stress and dance, and the kinds of relationships between dance and stress.

Chapter 1
In the Spotlight

Focus

At the outset, I will define what is meant herein by the terms *stress* and *dance*. Then I will turn to the manifold relationships between dance and stress, focusing in particular on some approaches involving dance that peoples have used to avoid and buffer stress. I must admit my bias in this regard. Dance has helped me to develop strength to ward off the debilitating effects of stress as well as to reduce its impact. Through dancing I have experienced catharsis, tension dissipation, physical and psychological relaxation, and euphoria. However, as the following pages will reveal, dance in its infinite variety is a multifaceted phenomenon. To be sure, at times dance itself may trigger stress for the doer or viewer. My Conclusion will offer some guidelines for dancing and the avoidance of harm. Along our path towards understanding the value of dance in stress management, those interested in the phenomenon of dance per se may find answers to some of their questions.

A number of the stress management techniques described in this book come from different cultures, past and present. Culture refers to the values, beliefs, attitudes, and learned behavior shared by a group and learned through communication. Individuals contribute to culture, which is a dynamic ever-changing phenomenon. For several reasons, a *cross-cultural perspective* is valuable.

3

First, I draw upon material on dance and stress from families, villages, and societies that seem, at first glance, to have little in common with what is found in modern society. Yet in our contemporary, pluralistic world we find vestiges of these traditions in homes, streets, and neighborhoods. History provides an enlightening record of where we have been and where we are. We find common underlying patterns as a result of diverse peoples' common humanity.

Second, a cross-cultural perspective helps us to increase our repertoire of the spectrum of possibilities from which we may choose. Through examining the dance practices of other societies, we can gain new insights and apply, with modification, certain approaches to our own situations. Not only does one generation pass down a cultural heritage to the next, but individuals also learn from other groups. A comparative perspective is often a mindstretcher, prejudice-dissolver, and taste-widener. Even though our social organization, cultural artifacts, and general technology have changed significantly over the millenia, there is little evidence that the human, as a member of a species with a psychobiological inheritance, has changed. We still refer to Plato and doctors find curative medicinal practices of isolated exotic people worthy of "civilized" people's attention. What works for one member of the human species just possibly may work in toto or in transformation for another, irrespective of the environmental complexity.

Third, a cross-cultural perspective can prepare health practitioners/clinicians/therapists to deal better with neglected or under-served diverse ethnic and socioeconomic populations, while recognizing underlying similarities among all groups. During the 1968 Joint Conference of the Research Department of the Postgraduate Center for Mental Health, the Committee on Research in Dance, and the American Dance Therapy Association, a number of clinicians commented on the fact that they were unable effectively to reach clients who were not middle-class white Americans. I discovered time and again in my various field research studies of social interaction that all people do not express themselves or interpret movement the same way.

For example, in an exploration of school children's social life in a multicultural, socioeconomically mixed elementary school, I asked boys and girls in grades two, four, and six how they can tell if a child feels different emotions (Hanna, 1982; 1988b). Several clues identified the same emotion. In answer to "How can you tell if a child is angry?" several children focused on arm-hand action and physical contact: "Sometimes they slug you," said a sixth-grade boy. A second-grade youngster put it this way, "They balls his fist—they pushing." The appearance of the entire body was a clue for other children: a sixth-grade girl remarked, "Sometimes they puff up." The stomping of feet also indicated anger. Children said the face attracted attention: "They roll the eyes at you, get all hunched up"; "When a boy gets mad, his lip start sticking out." Occasionally an expression intended to be friendly was interpreted otherwise, which triggered a fight.

Since the body is composed of universal features, most members of the Western medical and therapeutic professions that use dance in therapy erroneously assume that the body is experienced in a universal manner (cf. Manning and Fabrega, 1973). Similarly many professionals mistakenly believe all people experience the universals of time, space, and energy in the same way. However, assumptions concerning the biological and psychic unity of humans ignore the influence of cultural learning. Cultures, it should be noted, may be based on age, sex, ethnicity, race, occupational group, and so on. The handicapped, mentally disturbed, and mentally regarded may sometimes be conceived of as having their own cultures. Cross-cultural and social class problems are particularly evident in urban areas where most publicly and privately supported professional dance training and therapy occurs.

Because humans spin webs of significance from their own cultural perspectives, therapists need to understand how individual clients, as well as the cultures to which they belong, view the cause of a problem and the progress of its resolution. Movement should be seen in the context of how individuals learn to move and how appropriate the movement is according to their groups. Movements, usually possessing little meaning in and of themselves, reveal meaning only as the larger pattern of behavior of which they

are apart is identified and explained. The body has many components, each of which may send a different message.

It is, therefore, critical to know the cultural conceptions of educational and therapeutic approaches; the criteria for who participates
in dance, when, where, and how; and what movements are pre-
ferred, prescribed, and proscribed. This knowledge can determine,
for example, whether it would be preferable to opt for creative or
imitative techniques and individual or group interaction.

Resisting and reducing stress in many societies involves a mobilization of personal networks. Consequently, effective therapy may
require networks of persons who radiate outward from the ill person (family, friends, neighbors).

Fourth, a cross-cultural perspective may widen the understanding of how people constitute meaning in movement. Because there
are cultures in the arts, avant-garde participants may perceive images in abstract dance presentations that more traditional art audiences miss.

A case in point: at one of Douglas Dunn's dance concerts, a couple performed a duet. Spectators offered opposite views on
whether or not the dancers conveyed feeling in the dance before
the first intermission and how they felt in response to what happened on stage. Forty-six percent saw *no emotion*. People unfamiliar with abstract renderings or hostile toward them described the
movement as mechanical, stilted, robot-like, and computerized.
"It made me feel like I was watching androids or mechanical man-
nequins," said a respondent. Yet, other audience members perceived a wide range of emotions, although they differed in their
personal feelings in response to the same emotions. Forty percent
of the respondents observed *eroticism*, a rather strong emotion. A
male engineer perceived this feeling in the intertwining and roll-
ing of the couple on the floor, and he said it made him feel
"horny." Another person viewed the dancing as "X-rated." A male
lawyer saw ecstasy as the dancers were "lying as if spent," and he
felt "excited" (Hanna, 1983).

It is important to note that there are few statistically based and
analyzed control studies that demonstrate specific relationships
between dance and stress. However, compelling supportive case

material exists. Moreover, there is theoretical justification for the propositions about dance and stress. There are also scientifically documented bodily processes involved in human dancing that help us to understand the dynamics of how the dance-stress relationships work.

Concept of Stress

Subjective and Sociocultural Appraisal. Stress means different things to different people. I use pioneer Hans Selye's definition of stress: " 'the nonspecific (that is, common) result of *any* demand upon the body' be it a mental or somatic demand for survival and the accomplishment of our aims" (1980, p. vii). Stress is a response process that occurs when individuals have to cope with demands that require functioning above or below their habitual level of activity. A stressor indicates force that produces strain when a person is pushed to the outer limits of a particular adaptive capacity.

Of course, pressure is a matter of degree, and it is both subjective and objective as well as positive and negative. Moreover, internal and external predispositions or immunizing factors modulate the individual's response to strain. An individual may perceive stress without manifesting any objective, verifiable indication. Contrarily, a person may manifest stress and refuse to admit it, because admission would suggest self weakness or inadequacy.

Perception of stress depends on individuals' personalities within the context of their cultural and social groups. These shape individuals' values about life events and structure social interactions with people who may become either stressors or supporters. This variability means that some individuals are what in common parlance is referred to as "cool," not easily perturbed. Other people are short-tempered.

A situation that one culture deems stressful, another may take in stride. Loud noise, for example, may be comforting or distressing depending upon what people are used to. From infancy, Inuit Indians are accustomed to falling asleep easily in a noisy household. An outsider might find such a setting too stressful for a good night's sleep (McElroy and Townsend, 1979). Competitive, hostile environments tend to create tensions that cooperative, friendly settings preclude.

Causes. Causes of stress are a matter of how people respond to changing and, more importantly, conflicting demands in their lives. Potential stressors include transitions in the life cycle, its crises (especially divorce or a spouse's death), gender identity, residential relocation, education, work, and retirement; attitude and emotional reaction to injury and epidemics; inadequate resources; disjunction between aspirations and ability or opportunity; opposing political or religious values; family and community relations; natural disasters such as earthquakes, floods, and fires; ravages of war; discrimination; contact with another culture that rapidly and irrevocably changes a people's way of life through the introduction of new values and patterns of behavior or depletion of food sources, epidemics, war, genocide or confinement to reserves; and fears of nuclear holocaust, crash of the economy, overpopulation, and general unpredictability. In modern society stress often stems from doing things at odds with your feelings, sensing that you do not have enough time to do what you want, and feeling stretched while working at high gear. All illnesses cause stress.

Eustress and Distress. Stress may have positive results—that is, be eustress. It catalyzes adaptive, productive, creative efforts to solve problems. Moderate amounts of discomfiture are *alerting* and invigorating. A person who undergoes a stressful life event may, as a consequence, suffer no immediate disability or permanent damage but realize psychosocial growth. The stressor might stimulate the individual's commitment to achieving goals and induce healing processes.

Pursuing a passion for the glory of success and the potential for *euphoria*, some people deliberately *seek out stress* in such *challenges* as athletic competition or a dance career. Stress motivates these individuals to higher peaks of performance. Other people seek stress for therapeutic and religious reasons. Deliberately pushing the body and mind beyond normal limits through sensory overload to deprivation is a modality to experience a *vision* or mysticism.

There is another kind of positive stress. Dance with a sensory overload may induce stress which in turn brings on a state of resistance or strength to reduce other stressors, that is, a cross-resistance. During certain stress-inducing dances, participants may escape from the stresses of everyday toil for survival and achieve euphoria.

Negative stress, or distress, occurs when the body's defenses against the *harmful* effects of stress become overworked and exhausted. Stressors are accompanied by specific side effects that include feelings of frustration and resentment, emotional outbursts, muscular tension, violence, withdrawal, depression (generalized feelings of hopelessness, despair, sadness, or pessimism), anxiety (foreboding about impending disaster), nervousness, hand trembling, rapid heartbeat, shortness of breath, increased perspiration, high blood pressure, difficulty in swallowing, headaches, diffuse aches and pains in the joints, loss of appetite, fever, insomnia, skin eruptions, gastrointestinal disorder, thermal disturbances (icy hands despite heat, or hot body in a cold environment), lowered resistance to disease, and problems of concentration. Researchers have found that a host of more serious mental and physical illnesses plague stress-ridden individuals. Doctors have estimated that emotional stress and its accompanying muscular tightness may contribute to about 80% of back problems. Agoraphobia and its associated panic attacks, thyroid disease, diabetes, asthma, heart disease, cancer, and gastric and duodenal ulcers are also associated with stress. Periods of minor, chronic, or acute physical or psychological stress suppress elements of the immune system that defend the body against invading microorganisms like viruses, bacteria, and toxins (Glaser, 1986, and Kiecolt-Glaser, 1986).

On one hand, what appears to be a maladaptive response may reduce sociopsychological stress. On the other hand, what appears to be adaptive may be only the momentary escape during which an individual deals with the symptoms and not the causes of stress.

Body Mobilization. Selye called the three phases of the stress response pattern the *general adaptation syndrome* (1976). First, the body mobilizes to cope with irritation or harsh conditions in an *alarm reaction.* The body's defense during stress is to produce inflammatory hormones and then, in the second phase of the stress response pattern, the *stage of resistance*, to produce from the adrenal cortex anti-inflammatory hormones that limit the extent of inflamation against stressors and return the body to normal. The balance and interaction of these defense responses affect the relative resistance of the body to harm during the stress process. If a person continues to experience stress, the *stage of exhaustion* develops in which resistance declines. Stress alters the body's immune system and places an extra burden on the heart and blood vessels.

In the physical or psychological stress response pattern, other biological processes automatically prepare the body for defense. Cannon (1929; 1932) calls this action the *fight-or-flight* response. This syndrome does not require an emergency; indeed, everyday worries and pressures or extraordinary excitement may trigger the response.

Cannon's work, especially the notion of homeostasis between sympathetic and parasympathetic nervous systems, influenced Selye's early investigations. During the alarm reaction, the sympathetic nervous system goes into action in response to a stressor. It facilitates mobilization of adaptation energy and mental and muscular alertness in the form of biochemical substances.

Stress upsets the normal cycling of brain chemicals. *All* extreme emotions cause the brain to trigger a physiological reaction. Brain cells called neurons fire electrical signals stimulated by seeing, hearing, or smelling and associated thoughts. The brain then produces through the hypothalmus an excess of the corticotropin-releasing hormone (CRH), which sets off a series of chain reactions throughout the body, giving it increased speed and strength. CRH stimulates the pituitary gland to produce molecules of adrenocorticotropic hormone (ACTH). This chemical excess moves into the bloodstream to reach the adrenal glands atop the kidneys. The ACTH stimulates the adrenals to overproduce cortisol, another chemical, which signals other organs. Cortisol induces the formation and/or release from the liver of glycogen, which can be converted into sugar in the blood stream and thus provide more energy. The liver also burns protein for extra energy instead of converting it to muscle. At the same time, hormones mobilize fat reserves and release them into the bloodstream in the form of free fatty acids that the muscles can use as fuel. The immune system partially shuts down in preparation for possibly injury, so that the body does not overreact and attack itself.

Nerve fibers signal the adrenal gland to secrete the similar hormones epinephrine during fear and norepinephrine during anger. These two hormones speed up the heart to increase blood pressure and pump extra blood to the muscles and brain. Pupils of the eye widen as some blood vessels dilate. Other blood vessels supplying the stomach and intestine constrict inhibiting activity in these areas. In this way, the need for food is decreased, and the oxygen and blood supply to the brain and muscles for fighting or fleeing is increased.

The cascade of all these biological stress reactions may lead a person to experience increased euphoria and confidence or a vision.

After the sympathetic system action, the parasympathetic system begins to operate in order to conserve energy and rest the body. Pupils constrict, blood pressure and heart rate lower, and digestive processes resume. The kidneys excrete excess cortisol, epinephrine, and norepinephrine into the urine.

When a person neither fights nor flees because physical action in the immediate situation is inappropriate, biochemical elements of energy may remain in the body. For example, fats released that are not metabolized may be deposited in the internal lining of the arteries. Limited research suggests a repetition of such pattern of enduring stress may lead to atherosclerosis, a narrowing through obstruction of the arteries. This is one of several stress-related problems that contribute to cardiovascular diseases. Consequently, the mobilization capacity is likely to be maladaptive for individuals who do not use the energy generated. It can be released in physical exercise, including dance, varieties of which I will describe in this book.

Concept of Dance

On the basis of the views of various groups worldwide, my research observations of many dance forms, and a survey of the literature on behavior generally called dance, I think dance can be most usefully defined in the following way: human behavior composed (from the dancer's perspective, which is usually shared by other members of the dancer's culture) of purposeful, intentionally rhythmical, and culturally patterned sequences of nonverbal body movements other than ordinary motor activities, the motion (in time, space, and dynamics) having inherent and "aesthetic" value and transformative potential for the dancer and onlooker. Elsewhere I have discussed this conceptualization at great length (Hanna, 1979a; 1984; 1987d).

Physical Dimensions. The human body, instrument of dance, releases energy through muscular responses to stimuli received by the brain. The body or its parts contract and release, flex and extend, gesture and move from one place to another. The physical exercise of dance may be an end in itself, the purpose being the pleasure of doing. Or dance may be part of courtship, mating, healing, the promotion of solidarity and cooperation, or preparation for work or war, as in many non-Western societies in which dance served as military training. Dance serves a wide spectrum of purposes, including preventing and coping with stress.

Affective Patterns. The physical activity of dance may cause emotional changes and altered states of consciousness, flow, and secular and religious ecstasy. These changes are often stress related. Dance may increase one's energy and provide a feeling of invigoration. The exercise of dance increases the circulation of blood carrying oxygen to the muscles and the brain as well as alters the level of certain brain chemicals, as in the stress response pattern. Vigorous dancing induces the release of endorphins thought to produce analgesia and euphoria.

States of consciousness, always changing, range from tranquility to arousal, euphoria to anxiety. These states are the individual's perception of his or her own central nervous system. Altered states of consciousness create the feeling of a qualitative shift in thinking, disturbance in the time sense, loss of control, change in body image, perceptual distortion, change in meaning, sense of the ineffable, feeling of rejuvenation, and hypersuggestibility.

Csikszentmihalyi (1975) speaks of *flow*, a feeling of creative accomplishment and heightened functions. Flow elements include a centering of attention, loss of self-consciousness, sense of control, and the joy of taking action. Religious ecstasy involves a sense of shifting boundaries of time and consciousness, usually from the secular to the sacred.

Erik Bruhn, who for over 30 years represented the distillation of pure classical ballet, reached the height of euphoria four or five times in his career. "There have been certain moments on the stage where I suddenly had a feeling of completeness. . . . I felt like a total being. . . . It was a feeling of *I am*. At those moments I had the sense of being universal . . . but not in any specific form" (quoted in Gruen, 1986, p. 33).

Dances in communal settings often build up a spirit of elation that is infectious. The body is the first form of human power. Groups of people dancing together create a yet more powerful body. The year 1986 witnessed televised scenes of South African urban blacks dancing their protest against apartheid and white domination. A group often asserts a contagious force among individual dancers and spectators. Enveloping dancers in a close involvement, group performance may be ecstatic, a "communal sneeze" (catharsis, which I will discuss later), escape to a dream world (communitas), or supportive setting from which an individual temporarily obtains release from such involvement (detachment). The condition existing for one person in a group may be completely opposite to that of another.

Because dance is different in some ways from other aspects of daily life, its performance usually provides a change of life-space that differs from the workplace. In an atmosphere unlike the work environment, the dancer and onlooker may find a refuge for relaxation and nonwork kinetic thought.

Some cultures require temporarily changed eating patterns preceding dances such as rites of initiation or healing rituals, to further heighten an altered state of consciousness or religious revelation. Dance practices may alter blood sugar levels, which in turn affect how a person feels. The maintenance of a blood glucose level within certain limits is critical for the body (the brain consumes a major portion of glucose, roughly a fifth of the body's calories at rest). Fine hormonal regulation helps maintain the blood glucose level. Beta cells in the pancreas constantly monitor blood sugar levels and release the hormone insulin, the "fuel coordinator," accordingly. Without food or with prolonged dancing, glucose supplies in the circulation begin to dwindle and the low levels of insulin initiate the mobilization of stored fuels in the muscles. Because the muscles cannot convert glycogen into glucose for release into the blood, the muscle carbohydrate stores in one area are of little use for muscles elsewhere in the body. The liver acts as the major energy "transformer" and produces and releases glucose into the bloodstream by breaking down its stores and increasing the uptake of raw materials to produce glucose. If liver glycogen stores are depleted from prolonged dancing or low carbohydrate intake, and depleted fat stores through poor nutrition restrict the availability of free fatty acids for energy needs, the liver may not be able to meet the demands of a situation, and hypoglycemia may set in. Symptoms include sweating, fatigue, spasms, numbness, and palpitation.

Energetic dancing, high speed effort, sensory rhythmic stimulation in more than one sensory mode (kinetic and sonic action through musical accompaniment), and low-key dancing over long periods of time may also change the dancers' brain wave frequencies and adrenalin. These changes induce giddiness or other altered states of consciousness. The accumulation of by-products of muscular exertion in the blood results in fatigue and an oxygen debt (the inability of the body to take in as much oxygen as is being consumed by the muscular work).

Sometimes dancers may hyperventilate, or overbreathe. When people are anxious or excited, they breathe faster than normal. Consequently, they exhale more carbon dioxide, which changes the body's chemical balance. This change alters blood flow, the amount of circulating oxygen, and the way nerves and muscles work, leading to faintness, dizziness, and lightheadedness.

Cognitive, Nonverbal, Symbolic Communication. The cognitive dimensions of dance may also arouse emotions and contribute to altered states of consciousness, flow, and religious exaltation. We now know that the sensuous aspects of the dance experience do not exist apart form any mediation of ideas. Drawing upon the same cortical faculties of the brain that operate in verbalization, the dancer makes decisions about using his or her body in a particular way. Dance, as spoken or written language, is communicative behavior. We may think of dance as a text in motion, a visualization and embodiment of thoughts and feelings expressed or symbolized. People's thinking, through words or dance, about concepts, events, and feelings may be emotional.

It is important to distinguish the dance of humans from the dance-like movements of other animals or the spontaneous emotional kinetic expression of children. As humans evolved, the programmed action sequences (developmental instinctual behavior) characteristic of other animals tended to be replaced by actions in which cultural learning and individual purpose played a greater role. Consequently, in contrast with other animals and young children, more mature humans select action patterns. The basis for this contrast lies in the evolution of the human brain. It expanded in size and became restructured in the cerebral cortex to permit greater memory storage and multiple, fine perceptual discriminations, coordination, integration, and novel classification. Human evolution also led to increased dependency and socialization of offspring. These changes allow the transmission of a cultural heritage, which includes nonverbal communication. And within this domain lies dance. Notwithstanding individual creativity, a dancer's performance reflects a cultural heritage.

Following cultural rules, humans in their dances can voluntarily express or withhold emotions and ideas distanced in time and space from immediate stimuli. Using their bodies, dancers can choose rhythms with which to harmonize or counter. Their nonverbal movements are other than ordinary motor activities. A dance walk is not, for example, merely to move from one place to another but also to fulfill aesthetic values. Aesthetics, in a cross-cultural perspective, refers to notions of appropriateness and competency held by the dancer's cultural group.

Through dance, humans have the capacity to communicate abstract concepts, to project experience beyond their own, to alter feeling and thought and to transform them symbolically through various patterns. Such transformation occurs through different devices and spheres for sending messages, as I will point out later. The linquistic analogy may be helpful here. Dance is often less like prose than it is like poetry, with its suggestive imagery, rhythm, ambiguity, multiple meanings, and latitude in form. In a dance performance, as in spoken and written languages, we may not see the underlying universal and cultural structures and processes but merely their evidence. Structures are a kind of generative grammar, i.e., a set of rules specifying the manner in which movement can be meaningfully combined. Semantics refer to the meaning of movement, whether it is the style itself or some reference beyond the movement.

As in language (with its words, sentences, and paragraphs), dance has movement vocabulary, steps and phrases which may comprise realistic or abstract symbols and evoke an affective mood. It is important to note that dance can be symbolic even when a dancer intends no symbolic communication. From their own experience, spectators find associations in the visual images dancers frame for scrutiny.

Dancers are social commentators. Their performance may mirror what is in life, either as a validation or as a critique. Alternatively, dance may suggest what might be, through reversing usual actions, mocking the status quo, or presenting innovation. Whichever way, social dominance patterns in the broader society usually appear in the production of dance as well as the images of performance.

Assuming a communication intent, what contributes to received messages in the performer-audience exchange? It appears that shared knowledge and expectations are critical to getting an intended message. Understanding may vary according to knowledge about dance: being an outsider to a society, a knowledgeable observer, or insider (including a dance expert such as a critic, guru, movement analyst, a dance teacher, a choreographer, a dancer as executor of movement, or a dancer as creative interpreter of movement).

The importance of dance in communication lies in the fact that there are alternative ways of knowing, glossing experience, and different types of communicative competencies, including bodily kinesthetic competence, as Gardner points out (1983). Some people are imagers. Furthermore, Gazzaniga argues that "the normal person does not possess a unitary conscious mechanism where the conscious system is privy to the sources of all his or her actions . . . the normal brain is organized into modules. . . . All except one work in nonverbal ways such that their method of expression is solely through overt behavior or more covert emotional reactions" (1985).

Germaine to the cognitive dimension of dance is the fact that the dancer in contemporary America is the image of eternal youth; onstage the individual's dream life and culture's myth life merge. The physical realism of dance, therefore, may camouflage an appropriation of a dreamlike symbolic language. Dance transforms complex inner experience, desires, and feelings, and persuades people to accept other messages being conveyed.

Having introduced the scope of this book and presented the subjects of both stress and dance, I would like to consider now the kinds of relationships between dance and stress.

Chapter 2
Relationships Between Dance and Stress

Manifest and Latent Functions

In a discussion of dance and stress, the reader should bear in mind that dance can fulfill manifest and latent functions. Manifest are those behavioral consequences that are intended and recognized by the people involved, and latent are those which are not (Merton, 1957, p. 51). Dances simultaneously may have both functions. For example, a dance celebrating the birth of a child may be seen by a group to encourage the group's fertility, but the contribution of the dance to group solidarity or an individual's tension release may not be recognized. The latent meanings of a dance are deduced from sociocultural settings as well as from theoretical considerations that are more general, that is, in a wider setting than the experience one culture alone provides.

Relevant to this book is the concept of implicit intention (Dutton, 1977): the consequences that dancers do not recognize but take for granted; the consequences that dancers do not recognize in the same way as outsiders do but that may be equivalent; and the consequences that dancers do not recognize but are implied by the regular recurrence and systematic consequences of their behavior.

There are at least three key relationships between dance and stress to which I have alluded. Let me state these explicitly. (See Morgan, 1984, on physical activity and mental health.) The relationships may bear upon the dancer doing the dance or the viewer having empathy and vicarious experience. (Dancers may also be viewers when they move in unison with a group, perform before a mirror, or see themselves on film or video.)

One or more psychological processes may be involved in the dance-stress phenomena. Although various schools of psychotherapy and health promotion have defined these concepts within their respective theoretical perspectives of personality and human development, the concepts used follow general English usage unless otherwise specified (Fenichel, 1972; English and English, 1958; Harre and Lamb, 1983, present specialized definitions).

Dance and the Prevention of Stress

(1) Dance may be an activity that contributes to the prevention of stress, a kind of stress innoculation, through cognitive and/or physical action. The two actions are usually interrelated. Dancing develops enhanced well being and higher tolerance levels to stressors.

Cognitive Process. (1a) Dance may recount through the imagery of kinetic discourse *anticipated events* that have potential anxiety or feared consequences. Presenting these imaged concepts or narrative may enable individuals to play with them, to distance them, and consequently make them *less threatening*. This action is like a rehearsal. Failure is also acceptable and benign, because dance, after all, is only play and without the impact of real life failure. If one does not like the performance scenario, another can be created.

Past and current experiences may also be danced. These imaged kinaesthetic expressions have the potential to move an individual to evaluate problems, consider resolutions, and act in a constructive way outside the dance setting.

The effect of an activity depends in part upon the *meaning* a participant attributes to it. Dancing may give an individual a sense of *self-mastery* through being in charge of the body and its actions, physical health, and appearance. The sense of self-mastery contributes to a positive self-perception, body image, and esteem. Religious belief determines *possession* and *trance* states achieved through dancing that causes an excitation of vestibular apparatus and an altered state of consciousness with symptoms of dizziness, spatial disorientation, hallucinations, and muscular spasms. Trance is a sleeplike state characterized by reduced sensitivity to stimuli with the loss or alteration of knowledge of what transpires. Contact with supernatural entities through possession and trance provide guidance for individuals and their communities.

Physical Behavior. (1b) Dance's contribution to physical *fitness* may counter the negative effects of stress and illness. Before the birth of Jesus, Plato argued in the *Republic* that the soul or spirit benefits from regular vigorous activity. Effects of such movement have been mentioned as beneficial by philosophers from Aristotle to Freud. Exercise reduces the risk of certain life-threatening diseases. The Harvard University alumni study under the direction of Dr. Ralph S. Paffenbarger, Jr. (1986) showed that moderate exercise could help prevent heart attacks, and lower blood pressure and total serum cholesterol, while increasing the levels of the protective cholesterol carrier high-density lipoprotein (HDL). Physically active women are less likely than sedentary women to develop breast cancer. Exercise also helps to ward off adult-onset diabetes, strokes, and depression.

Dancing conditions the individual to be able to reduce, eliminate, or avoid chronic *fatigue* or lessen the impact of acute fatigue that are symptoms of stress. A sense of invigoration is experienced through the increased flow of oxygen delivered to the brain and other body tissues. Some dances have aerobic patterns, movements that stimulate heart and lung activity for a sufficiently long period to produce behavioral changes in the body. Regular aerobic exercise makes the body work more, demand more oxygen, and use it more efficiently (Cooper, 1970). When the body uses oxygen efficiently, it requires less oxygen for a given amount of work. One's aerobic capacity depends on the ability to rapidly breathe large amounts of air (efficient lungs), forcefully deliver large volumes of blood (powerful heart), and effectively deliver oxygen to all parts of the body (effective vascular system).

The maintenance or restoration of an optimal level of physical fitness can contribute to the overall quality of the later years of an individual's life. *Aging* is a form of stress in the sense of the individual's loss of ability to adapt to the environment. There is a decline in elasticity of the major blood vessels, increase in resting pulse and blood pressure, degeneration of cardiac structures, loss of muscular and skeletal strength, decreased flexibility of joints comprised of cartilage, ligaments, tendons, and synovial fluid, slower reaction time, reduced clear thinking, and greater susceptibility to depression. Aging in cultures with limited expectations and roles for the elderly is often accompanied by melancholy, crankiness, and loss of self-satisfaction with one's looks.

Aerobic dance ameliorates some effects of aging and minimizes its discomfort through building fitness and endurance. Dance with calisthenics builds coordination, agility, and muscular strength in the limbs and torso (Brody, 1986b). Moreover, exercise helps prevent osteoporosis, a disorder in which bones lose calcium and become brittle. This disorder causes more than one million "spontaneous" fractures a year in people over 45, especially postmenopausal women. Inactivity is thought to be one of the contributing causes of osteoporosis. "Bone adapts, like any other body tissue; when stressed it hypertropies, when unstressed it atrophies" (Smith and Serfass, 1981, p. 179; Montoye, 1983).

Dance may prevent *premenstrual* discomfort. Some women experience one or more emotional, physical, or behavioral symptoms during the week or two prior to menstruation (irritability, anxiety, fatigue, depression, bloating and weight gain, breast tenderness, headache, cravings for particular foods, and insomnia).

✘Inherent in the exercise of dance without injury, physical disability, or psychological tensions (emanating from, for example, confronting sensitive themes in dance or experiencing stage fright as described in Chapter 8 and 9) is a natural *tranquilizing* effect. This may improve a dancer's problem-solving capability.

Expulsive of tension build-up, dance is a release that wards off the harmful effects of stress. The Dogon of Mali describe the rapid *gona* dance movement "as a relief, like vomiting" (Griaule, 1965, p. 188). Lambo, an African psychiatrist, described African dancing with the rhythm, vigorous movements, their coordination and synchronization, as inducing some degree of catharsis. The Greeks, too, spoke of dance and catharsis, a concept used in psychoanalysis to refer to the first step in understanding and eliminating underlying conflict.

Catharsis (also known as abreaction) in dance is a complex physical-cognitive process of recollecting and releasing past repressed emotions and tensions and thereby coming to terms with them. The process encompasses experiencing anxiety or conflict and then releasing energy and frustration—discharging distressful emotions in a substitution for action against the source of the problem (cf. Scheff, 1977). *Insight,* understanding and evaluating one's own mental functioning (including recognizing the irrationality of some of one's impulses) to bring about psychological change, is often a concomitant of catharsis. Lambo (1965) believes the essential psychological function of dance is the prevention of depression and of accumulation of other psychic stresses.

Nearly everywhere, dance, especially for recreation (ostensibly the most common kind of dance), is likely to be cathartic. A pleasurable expenditure of energy, it is movement differing from everyday behavior and its associated pressures.

Rapid motion in dance is especially *intoxicating,* altering "the state of consciousness, facilitating an orally regressive state of perception and feeling tone without attendant loss of acuity in intellection . . . which gives the feeling of bliss and elation" (Safier, 1953, p. 242). *Regression* refers to a return to earlier and less mature behavior or a manifestation of primitive behavior irrespective of the person's earlier behavior. Dancing may be *sublimation,* a redirection of energy belonging to a primitive expression into new, noninherited channels. Vertiginous, spinning and turning, movements lead to release and altered states of consciousness, which may clear the mind of distractions and bring about insight into one's self and community.

Vigorous dancing is linked with a sensation of well-being and increased self-esteem (Morgan, 1985). "Theoretical, correlational, retrospective, epidemiological, and experimental evidence suggests that vigorous physical activity, both acute and chronic, is *associated* with improved *affective states*" (Morgan, 1984, p. 142).

People dancing in warm, humid climates may experience simple heat exhaustion that results from diminished cardiac output as a consequence of increased blood flow to the muscles and skin. The result may be a feeling of dizziness or fainting (syncope) accompanied by a rapid pulse and often cool skin (Lamb, 1978, p. 283). Coupled with religious beliefs of spiritual possession, this experience appears to be associated with trance states that may serve to prevent stress.

Dancing has become part of health promotion or wellness programs. Business organizations concerned with cutting absenteeism and boosting the productivity and morale of their staffs have found sponsorship of these plans to successfully meet their goals. For example, the Johnson and Johnson company learned that its wellness program paid for itself through lower employee hospitalization costs and a 13 percent decrease in sickdays (Vogel, 1986).

Dance as a Response to Stress

(2) Dance is a remediative intervention to cope with stress. In this case, dance often functions in the same ways that it does to prevent stress. For example, dance discharges repressed aggression, provides a sense of mastery which causes a corresponding change in self-perception and self-esteem, and induces possession and trance. However, dance as psychological treatment is similar to other treatments that work well for some people who have specific problems under particular conditions.

As a response to stress, dance has these three manifestations: confrontation with stressors to reduce stress, diversion from stress, and relaxation of stress-induced muscle tension. All three patterns to cope with stress may involve catharsis as well as other processes.

Reduction of Stress through Confrontation With Stressors. (2a) Many people in the United States have developed a dislike for the stresses of modern society characterized by the technological post-industrial revolution of mechanization and impersonality. Some of these individuals confront the stressors by turning to dance perceived as a pristine human sentient phenomenon, a basic form of *expression* and *communication*, and an ennobling patterning of thought, feeling, and physical action that is under the individual's own control.

Because the non-dance arts in the mid 20th century centered on form and abstraction (with the human body appearing, if at all, disembodied and rootless), dance may have come into its own, in part, to meet the need for the aesthetic presence of the whole human body, self-exploration, and self-definition. The "lived-in body" (Serlin, 1985), even when presented in "abstract" formalist dance, symbolically sustains people's power in our mechanized society. Through dance training and practice an individual marshals power to discipline the instinctive and culturally-patterned movements of the body. As a result, the dancer gains control over the body and freedom to use it in a particular way. Dance achievement testifies to *self-control*, dominance, and ascendance, comparable to the human conflict with nature found in bullfighting. Consistent with the Enlightenment ideal that the arts be instruments in controlling nature, dancers shape the rhythms of life and make the difficult look simple in testament to human competency and potential.

Stress-induced mental illness (conceptualized as the breakdown in an individual's adaptation to the environment that creates subjective distress and objective disability, the result of disharmonies within persons and between them and their societies, and the expression of disorders of communication based on past experience) requires communicative modalities as the major redressive tools (Frank, 1973, p. 318). This viewpoint means that Western *dance therapy*, discussed in Chapter 11, in confronting stressors must focus on individuals as well as their past and present close interpersonal relationships. In many cultures dance responses to deal with stress convey messages and the production and performance involve the person's *family and community*. (See earlier discussion of the affective impact of group dancing.) Frank believes that "no form of American psychotherapy can approximate the influencing power of [non-Western and nonindustrial] healing or thought reform [education]. . ." (See Dow, 1986.)

By projecting their problems in the dance, individuals may be "working through" their difficulties. In this process, often under the guidance of a healer, either a shaman, deity in the guise of a possessed dancer, or Western dance therapist, an individual faces the same conflicts repeatedly until able independently to face and master challenges in everyday life. Distancing or holding up a problem to scrutiny allows evaluation and possible resolution. The dance is potentially a creative way of dealing with conflict, learning about the self, and gaining insight.

Diversion from Stress. (2b)Besides portraying a problem in dance in order to manage it, another way of responding to stress is trying to eliminate the difficulty by temporarily *escaping* from or transcending it. Vigorous or continual dancing can, for physiological and psychological reasons already mentioned, lead to an *altered state of consciousness*, flow, catharsis, physical exhaustion, and euphoria. Many societies recognize the empirically-supported supposition that physical exercise can alter psychological states. Contagious affect among dancers, musicians, and observers enhances distraction from stress.

As have many people, I have experienced elation through dancing, both when I was in a good mood and when I was in a state of mild depression or emotional upset from a failure or misfortune. I had the sensation of soaring, being on a "high" (similar to the euphoria from ingesting alcohol or LSD [lysergic acid dyalmathide in an experimental setting]), having light limbs, and feeling energy and power.

Enveloping oneself in dancing may serve as a diversion from stressful situations. Dancing may provide a "time out" from anxious thoughts like the relief one finds in meditation. The rhythmic motions of aerobic activity may trigger mechanisms similar to centering devices in meditation. Moreover, the activity of dance itself may substitute for negative stress-related habits or catalyze a different attitude toward one's situation.

State anxiety, a transitory condition of foreboding about an impending disaster that may be real, imaginary, or even unknown, responds to habitual aerobic activity. Strenuousness, which varies from person to person, is a major determinant in the response. But twenty minutes of sustained heavy breathing is minimum (Berger, 1984, p. 139).

Various endorphins (beta-endorphin and beta-lipotropin) produced by the brain, anterior pituitary gland, and other tissues and released into the body as a result of the physical activity of dancing can be morphine-line in *reducing* the perception of *pain* and producing a state of euphoria. Vigorous activity seems to make moderately depressed or anxious individuals feel better.

Dance, like other forms of intensive physical activity, "often provides a healthy *fatigue* or distraction which may abate a temporary rage crisis and thus allows more *enduring personality patterns to regain* ascendancy" (Munroe, 1955, p. 630).

Relaxation of Stress-Induced Tension. (2c) Research suggests that tension reduction following exercise lasts longer than "passive" therapies such as meditation and distraction (Morgan, 1985, p. 96). It may be that dance increases the levels of brain norepinephrine or serotonin, or both. These chemicals drop with stress-induced depression.

Dance may fulfill the prescription for aerobic exercise as part of premenstrual syndrome therapy. Not only does aerobic type dance have a *tranquilizing* effect that improves the ability to cope with stress, but it also helps to reduce body fat, which in turn lowers the amount of estrogen the body produces (Brody, 1986a).

In stress reactions, excess unused energy released by sympathetic nervous-system action may produce muscular or nervous tension. Emotional tension from any source tends to locate in the muscles and tighten them. If stress indications become habitual, they tend to cause the muscles and tendons to shorten and thicken. The physical exercise of dance can provide remedial neuromuscular action by *lengthening* and relaxing the *muscles*.

Counterindications for Dance as a Response to Stress. (2d) There are situations in which dance as an intervention treatment might be counterindicated for the same reasons that running, another aerobic form of exercise, might be counterindicated (Sachs and Buffone, 1984). For a patient with severe depression and a fragile ego, a failure in the dance experience might precipitate an intensive depressive episode or a suicidal gesture. Obsessive compulsives, anorexics, bulimics, and competitive workaholics might turn dancing into a destructive experience. The conclusion to this book has a section on guidelines for dance, both prescriptive and proscriptive, including warning signs where dance is counterindicated.

Dance and the Induction of Stress

(3) Not only can dance serve to resist or reduce stress, but it can also *induce* stress. The role of dance in stress patterns for amateurs and professionals depends on how the dancer perceives the experience, whether the act is enjoyable or not (the difference may not be noticeable to an outside observer). When a person's behavior is motivated by the enjoyment found in the behavior itself, self-confidence, contentment, and feeling of solidarity with others accrue. If external pressures or rewards motivate the dancer, the individual may experience insecurity, frustration, and a sense of alienation.

Danced Social Criticism and Sensitive Subject Matter. (3a) Perception and comprehension of the dance experience may lead to stress. The dance often provides a libel-free medium for social criticism, the target of which may undergo stress. Masquerades and possession dances may hide the identity of a dancer who transforms into another being and can speak with religious legitimacy. For Western dance as for other performing arts, the theater is an arena in which to play with sensitive issues without the penalties accruing to a person's expression of them in everyday life. Themes enacted in dance often bear upon the "raw" nerves of an individual's personal or group conflict to create stress for the dancer or onlooker.

Going to the Dance. (3b) Because many dance classes and theaters in the West are located in congested urban areas, the effort to physically get to and from a dance activity may be stressful. An individual may have to organize a busy life to fit it in. Fighting traffic to reach a studio or theater on time, getting something to eat on the way, and finding parking if one drives are part of the effort. If a person has children, arranging for a baby-sitter can present obstacles to overcome. Obtaining tickets can be difficult if a performance is popular; numerous phone calls must often be made because box office or ticket sales lines are busy. The high price of theater tickets may stress a spectator's economic resources. And then, if the spectator dislikes the performance, stress is compounded. During my study of the performer-audience connection, an audience member wrote on an interview form: "a rip-off . . . I think having to pay to see a performance like this is absolutely a SHAM! I am including my name, etc., for I wish to discuss this further and would like a refund." A couple complained to me that they had come for entertainment. It cost money, plus transportation expenses, and time, only for a disappointment.

Amateur Dancing. (3c) As in learning processes generally, some people may be *intimidated* by an instructor or fearful of making fools of themselves before the teacher or classmates. This is especially the case for amateur dancers. Sometimes in a social dance setting, an individual may experience rejection from potential partners, or partners may lack coordination or miscommunicate.

Professional Dance Career. (3d) Artistic development with a minimum amount of stress is an ideal that dance participants desire. Professional dance training may be stressful for the same reasons amateur dance learning may have such repercussion. In addition, the dance career has its own stressors. Besides being highly competitive, it is fraught with risks of physical and emotional injury, which may end one's professional life. In some technically demanding dance genres, for example, ballet, dancers must continually work their bodies far beyond normal use. Many dancers suffer performance anxiety, what is referred to as stage fright. Because contemporary dancers are expected to be thin, individuals who lack the good fortune to have the body metabolisms that enable them to eat whatever they fancy without gaining weight often experience stress associated with dieting and being rejected for roles because of overweight. Anexoria and bulima are eating disorders found among dancers (Vincent, 1979; Kirkland, 1986). Strong personalities sometimes experience stress from their roles as tools of the choreographer and consequently fear losing their individuality.

Dancers, especially in ballet, must cope with a short performance career and then a transition to a new career. Due to the physical demands of contemporary dance technique, one is bodily "old" by 30. Not having enough weeks of performance to be eligible for unemployment, low salaries, no savings, problems of obtaining insurance coverage, and touring create stress for many dancers. Teachers and company directors face the difficulty of finding spaces for training, rehearsal, and performance in times of rising rents at the same time that performance itself is limited in its productivity. Another stress factor is the conflict between the economic dilemmas and artistic goals of dance companies.

Dance Therapist Disregard for Cultural Values. (3e) Dancing in a therapy session in which the therapist disregards cultural values may also be stressful (Foulks et al., 1977). For example, dance therapy training is primarily Western-based and emphasizes individual self-expression in dance. By contrast, some groups find individuality antithetical to their value systems, in which the group acts in unison and the individual does not stand out. Anglo-Americans value each person shaping his or her own destiny and consider self-actualization for each individual unlimited. Many American Indian groups, however, value anonymity—accepting group sanctions and routinized patterns. Spanish-Americans tend to esteem routinized life and obedience to the will of God. Emphasis on autonomy and self-actualization (self-fulfillment in separation from external forces) may conflict with a high value placed on group solidarity and conformity in the culture of poverty among Afro-Americans. Moreover, the emphasis may appear to promise more than an individual can realize given the constraints of the broader society and economy.

If a people believe the cause of stress is external to the self, the therapist needs to ascertain what are the perceived boundaries of the self. If illness is punishment for transgression, then it is necessary to understand what is considered deviance and what amends should be made. If disease is believed to result from sin, then expiation is necessary for a cure.

In a comparison of styles of interaction, Farrer (1976) examined Anglo and Mescalero Apache Indian patterns and concluded that teachers—and I would add therapists—might provide familiarity and security for the Mescalero by drawing upon their cultural patterns. These change agents could provide role models for learning-by-observation rather than calling out rules, as in Anglo culture, use the disciplinary tact of removing an offender from the group rather than reprimanding the person verbally, permit physical closeness and group work among relatives rather than have individual activities, and organize people in circles rather than rows and rectangular shapes.

Mexican-Americans have distinct notions about styles of behavior in therapy. Curing behavior is expected to involve direct eye contact, rapid diagnosis, religious sanction, appreciation and respect for the patient's self-diagnosis, respect for the patient's beliefs, minimal physical contact, treatment in the family context, and consideration of male dominance over the female (Madsen, 1973, pp. 89–96). These notions are usually counter to Anglo practice. Thus its success in serving Mexican-Americans is minimal.

Catalysts for the use of dance in therapy vary among groups that are often thought of as homogeneous in their way of life. Illustratively, among the southwest American Indians, the Apachean and Pima peoples hold ceremonies when stressful conditions occur. Most of the Navajo Indian dances are prayers to cure a particular person's illness (Fergusson, 1931, p. xxi). On the other hand, the Pueblo groups have calendrically-set ceremonials intimately involved with the creative cycle, production of rain, and concepts of like-cures-like (as in sympathetic magic). Indians on their reservations use their traditional methods of dealing with stress. However, Indians in urban areas, who have taken on many of the "white man's ways," might better respond to Western therapies that bear similarity to their respective traditional ways: individualistic and situationally determined; or group and calendrically-set sessions.

Caveat

The dance-stress relationships—preventive, remedial, and inductive—are not, it should be noted, mutually exclusive. Some dances are prophylactic and may also be performed in a crisis situation to reduce, escape from, or eliminate stress. The same dances may for some individuals under specific conditions induce stress. Participants in the same dance may have different experiences. The reason dance in one case may induce stress and in another resist or reduce stress is related to views about the body and dance, to personality, and to situation of time, place, and pervading cultural and social context.

Types of Stress Management Approaches

The means of preventing and managing stress are variable and even contradictory. Stress may produce a nonpathological *cross-resistance*. The treatment for one stressor may increase the body's resistance to other stressors.

Some religious groups have set calendrical rituals and other rituals that come into play with specified crises that help followers avoid stress or react to stress in a constructive manner. There are approaches that involve action; others require stillness. The sacred and secular often intersect in healing techniques. Various types of stress management approaches are not always explicitly named as such. For example, participants in *religious rituals* that help people cope with stress may see these actions only as practices prescribed by belief systems related to supernatural entities. Followers of a *secular lifestyle* that serves to resist or reduce stress, and sometimes to escape it, may not be aware of such benefit.

Another kind of stress management program is *secular therapy*, which is rooted in ritual dance practice and shares common patterns with it. The shaman or medicine person in non-Western dances is an avatar of the dance therapist. Within the secular therapy type of stress management approach, there are two prominent models, human potential and medical. The latter has two different orientations.

In the *human potential model* the therapist helps the "healthy" individual to realize her or his own self qualities. Self-actualization refers to self-fulfillment and self-expression, and attainment of autonomy from external forces. The existential, humanistic psychologies are not concerned with disability but humankind more broadly.

The human potential model is similar to the *wellness*, or *holistic* health, *medical* model. Herein all aspects of the human being—mind, body, and soul—are viewed as related and essential to the other. It is in the balance of these in relation to an individual's environment that a state of wellness exists. The approach has roots in ancient and non-Western health methods. Hippocrates and Galen, Greek physicians, had recognized the value of exercise. By the time of the Renaissance, nutrition and exercise were thought to be ways humans could wrest control of their destiny from God's will. In a wellness model, some decision-making and responsibility rests with the client.

In contrast with the human potential or wellness model, the *typical medical model* assumes the client is ill and the therapist attempts to diagnose and heal the individual by aiding him or her to cope with the specific pathology. This model is related to the paradigm shift to Rene Descartes's dualistic philosophy, which had effectively separated the concepts of mind (and spirit) and body. The medical model is most relevant to the severely ill and mentally retarded.

Note that individuals may participate in these programs in a variety of ways: sequentially, at one time or another, or simultaneously in one or more.

Styles of Intervention in Stress Situations

The styles of intervening in stress situations are variable. *Autogenic*, or self-conducted, styles mean that the individual takes the initiative in some way, whether it is to meet one's god through dance, take a dance class, dance spontaneously, or visit a dance therapist. The individual maintains decision-making authority and responsibility for action. In *directive* styles a member of a society, such as family, priest, or therapist who observes stress-ridden behavior, will direct, or induce, the individual to act in a structured way toward specific goals. Another approach to stress intervention is *evocative* therapy, which helps people modify their behavior by indirectly creating favorable conditions for modification but eliciting their self-reflection and leaving change up to them.

More than one style of intervention may be operative at the same time. Each style may involve *interpretation* based on the therapist's theoretical system of psychology whether it is expressed in terms of cosmology and ancestor honor or Freud's ego and id.

Dance Genres Associates with Stress Reactivity

Not only are there variations in the kinds of relationships between dance and stress, types of stress management approaches, and styles of intervention in stress situations, but there are also different dance genres associated with stress reactivity. In the literature, one finds the oppositions of primitive versus theater, classical versus folk, social versus ethnic, ballet versus modern. The terms used are variously defined. Moreover, the categories often blur because of borrowing. For our purposes in discussing dance and stress, I will comment on several genres.

Ritual dance is an extraordinary event involving stylized, repetitive behavior. It may include practices of magic (sacramental utterances, exorcisms, curses, and blessings that are believed to set in motion some supernatural entity or transcendent power), prayer, and sacrifice. The concept of adaptation is immanent in dance vis-à-vis the supernatural. The function of adaptation is to link a social system and its environment, specifically, in this case, extracting goods and services from the supernatural environment for the society. Dance is sometimes part of religious expression to worship or honor the deities, conduct supernatural beneficence, effect change, embody the supernatural through an inner transforma-

tion and personal possession or through an external transformation as in a masquerade (Hanna, 1987a; 1987d, ch. 5; 1988a).
Steeped in religion, these dance practices bring to life the imaginary work of the invisible supernatural.

There are distinctions in ritual dances based on the kind of participation that is involved. Some dances are dancer-initiated. In
contrast with the dancer intentionally doing, the dancer may be becoming, that is, acted upon by the supernatural. Ritual dance, as
with totemic ideas and myth, appears to be part of a cultural code
enabling the human being to order experience, account for its
chaos, and explain affective and cognitive "realities." Coupling the
hedonic and cognitive, dance has the power to create a second
world, one of virtual time and space.

Dance is *ethnic* when it is explicitly linked to the sociocultural
tradition of a group with a sense of identity based upon origins
(an ethnic group's members constitute part of a larger society).
Ethnic dance is *folk* when it is a communal expression; folk dance
need not be ethnic, but both may be social, ritual or theatrical
dance. The context of a dance clarifies its type and whether it is a
first or second existence folk dance. A first existence refers to
"dance as an essential part of life," whereas a second existence refers to a revival or arrangement, perhaps a stage performance
(Hoerburger, 1965). The Russian Mosieyev Dance Company presents folk dances, but it certainly is considered theater dance. An
ethnic group in the United States may alternatively perform its
dance in a member's home at a holiday, as a social dance, or in a
theater for a heterogeneous audience. The lack of clear-cut dance
categorizations also appears in the view of ballet as ethnic dance
(Kealiinohomoku, 1969–70).

A key purpose of *social* dance is to provide the opportunity for
people to get together and interact. This genre includes popular
dance (common in the dominant culture in a heterogeneous setting), ethnic-folk, second existence folk, and some forms of
dance therapy.

Exercise dance refers to aerobics dance, jazzercize, and other
forms of bodily exertion that incorporate simple contemporary so-

cial dance-like movement patterns with musical accompaniment to make physical fitness activities more enjoyable.

Theater dance includes forms of dance that require specialized training and are presented onstage for an audience. Thus, ballet, modern (the rebellion against classical ballet heralded by Loie Fuller, Isadora Duncan, Ruth St. Denis, and Martha Graham), postmodern (the reaction to modern dance led by Merce Cunningham), jazz, tap, and Broadway musicals. Theater dance has limited audience participation; the spectator is distanced from the dancer.

Therapeutic dance activities depend upon the client's movement skill and vocabulary. Sometimes dance therapy uses only body movement and would not be recognized as dance per se by the average person in the United States.

Having presented some dance genres that are involved in stress management, and having noted that the categories are not clear-cut, we should be aware of the processes of change that have contributed to this phenomenon. Dance always transforms and may fulfill different functions at different times. People, as noted earlier, borrow from each other. Sometimes dances are imposed.

Now we will turn to dance-stress illustrative cases. The approach is to draw upon ethnographic, clinical, historical, and experimental research and to present a brief or longer discussion depending upon the available data in a given area.

PART II

Illustrative Historical and Non-Western Dance-Stress Relations

This section looks at dance practices related to stress that come from cultures different from those generally assumed to exist in contemporary Western society. The illustrations of kinds of relationships between dance and stress drive from earlier times, non-Western cultures, and Western minority cultures, both past and present.

The examples in the next five chapters will provide a cross-cultural perspective that can lead to innovation in one's own life and culture, effectiveness in dealing with people distinct from oneself, and improved understanding of meaning in movement.

We see dance-stress relations in single or multiple manifestations, latent or manifest functions, and different patterns in the sequential development of an event. Causes and symptoms of stress vary, as do the styles of stress management. Chapters 1 and 2 presented a theoretical framework for dance and stress. Although the typology of relationships is based on a survey of case material, the cases do not always fit neatly into one or another of the categories. Consequently, the following chapters are organized in terms of illustrative examples of dance and stress that cluster by specific mode of action or problems addressed: meeting the supernatural (Chapter 3), taking action in other religiously-motivated ways (Chapters 4 and 5), resolving conflicts in the secular arena (Chapter 6), and confronting political and economic changes stimulated by culture clash through old or new dance group patterns (Chapter 7). Ritual, social, and ethnic dance genres are described.

Some themes will reoccur in the chapters of Parts II and III. Death, for example, is a universally stressful event that people attempt to cope with in religious dance practices as well as secular dance. Feared not just by individuals but by societies, the cessation of life wrenches and dislocates part of the fabric of social relationships. The more important the person, the greater the number and range of ties are snapped. People must reorganize themselves after the demise of one who was at the center of a cluster of social relations. The death of others holds intimations of our own mortality and creates other kinds of anxiety and fear.

Contemporary psychologists recognize the need for bereaved individuals to have some help for a year or more in dealing with grief, coming to terms with the loss of someone close. We see ourselves reflected in the daily response of our partners. The mourning process involves both the mind and body. Stress is commonly marked by denial, anger, degrees of depression, and eventual acceptance.

People can "get stuck" in bereavement-linked depressions. The stress of bereavement tends to be disruptive to one of the body's basic systems of stress regulation, namely, the hypothalamic-pituitary adrenal (HPA) axis that is activated in the face of a threat of danger (Rovner, 1986). Therefore, remedial action is needed.

Chapter 3
Meeting the Gods and Demons to Cope with Stress

Praise and Appeal

Religious belief systems often have explanations for stressful events and behavior. The gods may be considered to cause famine; demons, witches, and spirits to make people ill or difficult to get along with. Dance is frequently part of a general ritual scene, social milieu, and specific ritual practices that are presumed to appease the divinities or exorcise demons or malevolence caused by spirits. Dance may be prophylactic, honoring supernatural entities to preclude their angry creation of stressors for natural beings. Thus human honorific performance for the supernatural reveres, greets as a token of fellowship or hospitality, and shows respect. Dance may also be remedial. In this case the dance propitiates or beseeches the supernatural entities to change stressful conditions, or is expurgatory. Dance may also be a religiously sanctioned "time out" (even euphoric state) to gain relief from the stressful situation. In healing rituals, the shaman, priest or equivalent particularizes part of the mythic world for the patient.

There are numerous illustrations of religious dance practices that serve to resist or to reduce stress. The following techniques are stylistically autogenic. The Old Testament refers to rejoicing with a person's entire being. Thus the Jews dance to praise their God in sublime adoration and to express thanks for his beneficence. The Kalabari of Nigeria say that men make the gods great. Fervent dancing adds to a deity's capacity to aid the worshippers—and just as surely the cutting off of dancing will render them impotent or at the least break off contact with erstwhile worshippers (Horton, 1960). The Sandawe of Tanzania believe the moon to be a supreme being who is either beneficial or destructive. Identifying with the moon, the dancers adopt stylized signs of moon stances to metaphorically conduct supernatural beneficence. The moonlit erotic dance in which couples tightly embrace and mimic the act of fertilization is assumed to promote fertility (Ten Raa, 1969).

Dance may be a medium to reverse a debilitating condition caused by the supernatural. When the Gogo men of Tanzania fail in their ritual responsibility for controlling human and animal fertility, disorder reigns. The women then become the only active agents in rituals addressed to righting the wrong. Dressed as men, they dance violently with spears to drive away contamination (Rigby, 1966).

Other religiously motivated modes of action to cope with stress are possession, masking, and exorcism. These modes may occur independently or in combination. They involve several psychological processes, especially catharsis.

Possession

Through the dance, a person may *invite* possession by giving the self temporarily to a supernatural, and thereby achieve a consciousness of identity or ritual connection. Experiencing an inner transformation to embody the supernatural, the dancer performs identifiable and specific patterns and conventional signs communicating to the entire group present that the supernatural is enacting its particular role in the lives of humans. Thus fear of the supernatural entity's indifference is allayed.

Cult and brotherhood members, diviners, medicine men, mediums, and shamans are among those who invite the gods to possess their bodies. The possessed then act on another person's behalf. In the spiritualist sects such as the Umbanda, Candomblé, Tango, Quimbanda, and Catimbo in Brazil, participants temporarily es-

3. Meeting the Gods and Demons to Cope with Stress : 41

cape from daily worries and gain liberation from blocked emotional tensions (Akstein, 1973).

A Moroccan Sufi brotherhood, the Hamadsha, perform the *hadra* ecstatic dance in order to cure an individual who has been struck by the devil or possessed by one. The ritual helps to relieve anxiety, physical tension, and emotional stress (Crapanzano, 1973, pp. 195–210, 231–234). Cult members, bothered by paresthetic pains (feelings of numbness, prickling, and tingling), find relief and a sense of revitalization in the dancing and trance.

Attack by a *jinn* (spirit) causes facial or other paralysis, convulsions or sudden (hysterical) blindness or deafness. McElroy and Townsend (1979) note that "excessive anxiety and hyperventilation can cause these symptoms by raising the alkaline level of the blood higher than normal (respiratory alkalosis). People attacked by a *jinn* often recover from these symptoms overnight if they dance; however, they may experience aftereffects of stillness, and a lack of energy.

"Using our knowledge of the stages of alarm, resistance, and exhaustion, we can see that respiratory alkalosis and paralysis are an alarm reaction to the stressor of anxiety, a recurrent psychological feature of the Moroccans who belong to the Hamadsha. Through a variety of sensory overload techniques, the dancers induce stress, which brings on a stage of resistance to the initial psychosomatic illness of paralysis. The depression and temporary fatigue experienced after trance are analogous to the strain evidenced in the stage of exhaustion; since the initial stressor is removed, however, there is little serious danger that this strain will lead to permanent damage" (p. 295).

The dancers seek a good relationship with a *jinn*, usually the she-demon 'A'isha Quandisha. During the ritual she may emerge from the ground and dance alongside the human performers. She causes the dancers' heads to swell, their hair to stand on end, and their scalps to itch. Slashing her own head is an example to them. As the dance progresses, the participants become entranced and, in imitation of the saint Sidi Ali's servant, slash at their heads. The flow of blood is believed to calm the spirit. Certain of the

Hamadsha form teams that perform the *hadra* professionally for the stricken and the sick.

Among the Irigwe of Nigeria, the traditional marriage custom calls for both men and women to marry several spouses from different tribal areas and for the women to shift residence among husbands several times during the lifetime. Perhaps to relieve the tension "arising from their repeated separations from loved ones and to achieve social integration to compensate . . . for the repeated separations," Irigwe women often become possessed during spirit cult dances, "cry, speak in tongues, and flail about after the frenetic drumming, dancing, singing, and rattling leg irons had induced a dissociated state in them . . . giving vent without castigation to their repressed feelings" (Sangree, 1969, p. 1055).

In Korea, the most elaborate shaman ritual, the *kut*, aims to bring good fortune, to heal, or to send off the dead. Following a sequence in which certain deities appear, the dance is a means to invoke the gods and encourage their descent into the shaman. The female shaman (who outnumbers the male practitioner in male-dominated Korea), is a specialist for housewives who experience gender-related stress (Kendall, 1985). In essence the shaman gives a "women's party" by and for women. Claiming to see the deities and beckon them to speak through her lips, she puts on a particular god's costume. To drum accompaniment, the shaman sings an invocation and then with outstretched arms dances gracefully until a burst of drumbeats and a series of leaps reveal the descent of the gods. Kicks and flailing arms announce that the gods are strong.

After a few shamans have invoked several of the sponsoring family's household gods, the shamans rest. During this interval one after another of the women of the household and their relatives and neighbors puts on the shaman's costume and dances to receive her personal god.

In the *invasion* possession dance, often a metaphor and signal of social pathology or personal maladjustment, the supernatural being overwhelms an individual causing some form of malaise, illness, or personal or group misfortune. The dance exorcises the being, thus freeing the possessed individual and ameliorating the irksome situation. Meeting the wishes of a spirit as part of directive exorcism usually imposes obligations on the possessed's relatives.

Individuals may experience invited or invasion possession by a supernatural potency. For example, among the !Kung Bushmen of Namibia, prolonged dancing to women's song heats up and activates n/um, a therapeutic substance that resides in the stomachs of medicine men who are renowned dancers. These healers derive their power for remediation and protection from sickness and death through this overwhelming potency within their bodies that exudes in sweat. The ceremonial curing dance with the medicine that can be transferred from these dancers to patients is called for during crisis situations, and it will occur spontaneously for good measure.

This Bushmen healing dance is both a case of people escaping stress and seeking stress for religious therapeutic purposes. People come together as a unit to sing, clap, and dance. "They are doing something together that gives them pleasure. They are enlivened in spirit and body. . . . They are lifted out of the arduous unremitting search for food and out of the anxieties that fill their days" (Marshall, 1969, p. 12; Lee, 1967). The dancing may last from 12 to 36 hours with individuals participating in four- to six-hour shifts.

The stimulation of the physical movement, the constant rhythm of the music, sensory overload, hyperventilation in breathing, and autosuggestion facilitate trance. When n/um boils through the sensory overload of the curing ritual with its stress of excessive stimulation, the men enter an altered state of consciousness, which the Bushmen call "half-death" and we call trance. The !Kung experience dizziness, disorientation, hallucinations, and muscle spasms. We would normally view these symptoms as alarming evidence of illness (McElroy and Townsend 1979, p. 277). The medicine man "in trance absorbs the patient's disease into his own body and lets it run its full course inside his body" (Guenther, 1975, p. 162).

Contact with white immigrants from South Africa and black ranchers who settled in the Ghazi district was disruptive to the San Bushmen. They experienced unemployment, poverty, hunger, and new diseases as well as a self-degrading self-image. The prominence of suffering has led to the trance dancer's unprecedented social importance. In contrast with the hunting-gathering Bushman, the farming Bushman trance dancer assumes professional status and achieves wealth and prestige. Moreover, with heroic and mystic power, the dancer revitalizes the Bushman culture and self-image (Guenther, 1975).

In a number of Christian denominations, dancers during church services may become possessed through, as they say, "feeling the spirit." For example, the black American Pentecostal Church of Holy Christ in Pittsburg believes God is the Father of Christ conceived by the Holy Ghost, and born of Virgin Mary. Dying for the sins of humans, Christ went to Heaven to prepare a place for them and left the Holy Ghost for their comfort. On the day of Pentecost, the Holy Ghost descended to the apostles and gave them "quickening powers" with speaking of tongues, dancing, and other manifestations of spiritual possession. Dance is thus treated as a divine occurrence, a revelation of God to those upon whom he has bestowed the Holy Ghost (Williams, 1974).

At the Mt. Pisgah Missionary Baptist Church in Dallas, on the 25th anniversary of the Senior Men's Choir, I observed the fervor of the church service reach a high emotional pitch. Individuals in the pews shouted, "amen," "preach it honey," "yes sir," "get on with it." They cried, nodded heads back and forth, swayed sideward, raised their palms upward, shaked, clapped their hands, and danced to the accompaniment in a gospel rhythm (similar to the blues and boogie) of the choir, pianist, and organist. While dancing, some women collapsed into the arms of male ushers.

Masking

Sacred masquerade dances have stress-related features common to possession dances. Both forms of ritual dance allow people to separate themselves from a problem by distancing or diversion from stress. The elicited religious and spiritual direction provides sanction and legitimacy for secular actions and allows performers and audience members to transact social relationships less stress-fully than in everyday life.

Masquerade dances are part of a people's intercourse with the supernatural world. The dancer embodies a supernatural entity through invited *external transformation*. Beneath the mask, a dancer is believed to undergo change. Under religious auspices, the dancer is freed from everyday restrictions and consequently can present critical messages that might otherwise produce stressful social friction or hostility.

For example, the Nigerian Nsukka Igbo council of elders employed masked dancers representing an *omabe* spirit cult whenever there was difficulty in enforcing law and order (Tamuno, 1966). A Chewa man residing in his wife and mother-in-law may resort to the male masked *nyau* dance to mediate between himself and a mother-in-law whom he dislikes for making constant demands on him. When he dons his mask as the *chirombo* (beast), he directs obscene language against her and no action may be taken against him. In his mask he enjoys the immunity of *chirombo*. The mother-in-law usually reduces her demands after the dance (Chilivumbo, 1969). Here is a case of catharsis and working through.

Socially sanctioned ritual abuse with ribald and lewd movements and gesture in a highly charged atmosphere occurs in the Ivory Coast Bedu masked dance. The Nafana people believe that through these acts participants will be purged of whatever negative emotions they may harbor (Williams, 1968).

The similar contribution of the Dogon of Mali masked dance is discussed in Chapter 4.

Exorcism and Healing

Possession and masquerade dances may occur in tandem; that is, masked dancers may become possessed. In Sinhalese Buddhist healing rites the exorcist, in a directive and evocative style, attempts to sever the relationship between a patient and malign demons and ghosts in order to reduce or eliminate stress. Emotional tension builds up progressively in the exorcist's performance of various masked dance sequences. These generate power that reaches out and embraces and then entrances the healer and/or the patient. Their bodies become the demonic spirit's vehicle, constitute evidence of its control, and convince spectators of the need for a change in social relations that will transform the patient from ill to healthy. Exorcism works to build the ideal social hierarchical order. The dance is a public validation first that the patient has fallen under a demon's control and then that a cure has been achieved.

Kapferer (1983) describes the demon ceremonies, particularly the healing rite of the Great Cemetery Demon, performed in the vicinity of the town of Galle in the southern area of Sri Lanka. The chief participants are the members of the urban working class and rural peasantry. Associated with tradition, specifically the subordinate and weak Sinhalese of the era of colonial rule, the healing rite has a disproportionate number of women victims.

The Sinhalese view is that women are subordinate to men. Yet they" are also central in the cultural order and the most sensitive to disturbances in it" (p. 108). Exorcists appear in the guise of women in the main dance episodes. In this manner, "the dancers are understood to attract the demons to ensnare demons in their own demonic natural passion, and make them prisoners of their own lust. Exorcist female attire is symbolic of the mediation of nature and culture in the identity of the female and the vulnerability of women to the attack and control by the demonic. It is during the dance, held at a time when demonic power is in its ascendancy, that an exorcist-dancer will become possessed by the demon" (p. 106).

Transvestism is not the point. Rather, "the strength and authority of the male lies behind and within the female. During the dance, the demonic enters into the male body of a dancer dressed as a female. Trapped in a male body, which is also healthy and nonafflicted, the demonic can be controlled and expelled. The illusory, the play on appearances and form which is such a constant theme of major exorcisms, is thus present in the dress of the dancers" (p. 151).

Exorcists are from a special caste, *berava*. Students seek recognized exponents with whom they study. Apprenticeships begin as early as six or seven years of age. Instruction usually begins with the dance and then proceeds to the art of drumming, intoning mantras (spells), and singing. Exorcists assist each other with performances.

The exorcist discovers the malevolent supernatural agents involved in the illness and also uncovers the social events surrounding the patient and others that have exposed the patient to demonic attack or are indicative of demonic malevolence. "A disturbance of the body is also a disturbance of the mind, and *vice versa*" (p. 183). Stress is obviously a critical cause. Extreme emotional states, especially fear, but including anger, envy, jealousy, grief, and acute sexual desire are symptomatic of demonic illness (p. 50). Exorcists typically trace its onset to the patient's experience of sudden fright or fear, whether in dreams or mysterious figures in the night. The patient's experience may be autogenic in calling for help.

The decision to have an exorcism is not undertaken lightly. Moreover, demonic agency in illness can be dangerous to those beyond the patient. "Knowledge that an individual is a demonic victim can lead other members of a neighborhood to reduce their interaction with a patient and a patient's household" (p. 62). For the treatment, patients and their immediate family require the material support and cooperation of other kin and neighbors. In the case of Asoka's illness, the agreement achieved to hold the exorcism was more than a consequence of the severity of her physical symptoms. The decision reflected for her kin a set of social difficulties related to conflict over land and property that they were encountering (p. 71). Demonic attacks gain prominence in the context of disruption and fragmentation in the social order.

A spectacular combination of sound, song, smell, dance, and drama, the "show" of demonic behavior performed throughout the night makes manifest to the senses of patients and onlookers the "real" intention of demons, which then become accessible to remedial action. To disclose is to expose to therapeutic action, since the unknown is dangerous. Demons seek to hide themselves from "reality," from exposure of their true place in the cosmic hierarchy. When Mahasona is revealed in his masked representations, they can be humiliated, mocked into their proper place in the scheme of things and cease to be awesome. "Caught out," they have nowhere to go except into ridiculous disgrace.

When the demons are made inferior to humans and the divine through danced comic action, the fear and terror of the demons can be laughed away. Not only are demons subjected to ridicule, but in parallel fashion the structure and contexts of everyday life are also made light of. Exorcists and onlookers enjoin the patient to participate in the comic action. The humor is crucial to treating a patient, who is brought out of demonic obsession/possession and restored to the world of social relationships.

Exorcism restores the individual to a sense of well-being (p. 177). The process involves a distancing that allows individuals to stand outside their own subjectivity, constitute themselves as objects, and then reconstitute themselves in a state of well-being.

The dancing episodes and entrancement of the patient constitute evidence in the views of the exorcist and audience that the patient has fallen under the demon's control. With elaborate dance the exorcists win the confidence of observers in their skills to overcome the demon. The comic mocking signifies that the demons are denied a position of dominance, whereupon the patient has the opportunity to be identified as no longer subject to demonic attack.

Dance draws those who are attentive to it into the demonic and divine realm of its creation. The exorcists understand their dances to constitute the greatest elaboration of supernatural force (p. 192). Exorcists and onlookers believe the dancer become one with the forces they generate.

Kapferer explains, "The exorcism is held to honour the demons, and they are treated as if they are gods. They are given offerings which seem appropriate to the gods—incense is burned, flowers and foods . . . are given. But the incense has the smell of death and pollution even while flamed as fire it 'destroys' and repels the demons. The flowers are shredded and dead. The foods are cooked and mixed with pollutants such as oil, flesh, and blood. What appears as suitable for the gods is suitable only for demons. . . . But the demons in their acceptance of them become vulnerable to their own destruction. Like the gods, the demons are presented with ceremony . . . the magnificent dance is in their honour. But as they are called and celebrated, so are the gods, whose authority and purity will destroy, control, and repel the demons. In the dance and the dancer resides the divine. . . . The entire rite . . . can be seen as the elaborate springing of a demonic trap, a means for refixing the demons in a cosmic order which they have momentarily escaped" (p. 229). The demons are embodiments of the manifold dimensions of life's suffering and symbols of destruction of humans and an encompassing cosmic whole.

Commentary

In meeting the gods and demons, or their representatives, through the dance medium, individuals often resist, reduce or escape stress. In dancing to appease the supernatural, appeal to reverse a debilitating condition, or exorcise malevolence, performers may develop physical fitness to ward off the debilitating effects of fatigue, old age, and pressures of daily life. The ritual of healing, validated through the associated dance, serves to mediate through religious legitimacy the social relations that caused an individual distress or illness. Much of the dancing is cathartic, working through, and prescriptive. Dancing in possession permits a temporary euphoric state and escape from anxiety and depression. Religious beliefs sanction many behaviors contemporary research scientists have found to be effective stress management techniques.

Chapter 4
Expelling Stressor Spider Venom and Shaking Off Death, Sin, and Evil

History attests to dancing as a response to the stressors of poisonous spider bites, plagues, peril, pestilence, and sexuality—indeed, a wide variety of medical/psychological syndromes. In this chapter, four illustrative cases (tarantism, the Black Death, Ketjak, and Shaker dance) are presented. The cases are related to both religious and secular behavior. Although the dance-stress pattern may have a specific initial catalyst, the performance may encompass other stressors as well.

Tarantism

Tarantism, in which dancing plays a key role in expurgating the venom and curing the bite (real or imaginary) of a particular spider, is a hysterical phenomenon related to dancing mania (Russell, 1979). A demand for attention and an outlet for pent-up emotions are prominent features of all outbreaks in response to stress.

From Rouget's (1985) English summary of the literature on tarantism comes the following information. In a text dating from 1621 and quoted by E. de Martino (1966, p. 385), we learn that victims of the tarantula bite, "almost moribund because of the venom, moaning, anguished, agonizing, almost bereft of . . . [their] senses, external and internal," could return to their senses upon hearing the sound of musical instruments. Such individuals opened their eyes, pricked up their ears, rose, began to make slight movements with fingers and toes and then, keeping the rhythm of the melody began dancing with great liveliness, "gesticulating with . . . hands . . . feet . . . head, with all parts of [the] . . . body shaken in all of its limbs by the most varied agitations."

The prepossession crisis is not a unique event in the possessed person's life, we are told, but it is usually commemorated in annual recurrences. Collapse occurs before as well as after the trance. During the entire time that the tarantulee is entranced, the dance is intended to lead to collapse except at the end, when the person is granted "grace" (de Martino, 1966, pp. 68–73). The perpetual motion is critical in the resolution. The music with its rhythmical order unleashes "that most elementary sign of life which is movement, while, at the same time, the discipline of the rhythm prevents the movement from sliding into pure psychomotoric convulsions."

Each species of tarantula has its own special tune although the same dance is performed. A musical motto was a means of identifying the spider responsible for the possession. In the late nineteenth century, twelve different tarantella themes were used to diagnose Naples tarantulees. An ill patient did not know if she had been bitten by a tarantula or by a scorpion. So the musicians who had been summoned began trying out their themes. "At the fourth, the tarantulee immediately began to sigh, and at last, no longer able to resist the call of the dance, she leapt half naked from her bed, without a thought for conventions, and for three days kept up a sprightly dance, after which she was cured" (de Martino, 1966, p. 160). The possession trance is a change of identity that is recognized by everyone through the dance.

A variant of tarantism appears in Sardinia. Here the mythical creature, the *argia*, causes the patient's poisoning. This creature "is categorized under three distinct species, the nubile, the wife, and the widow, and the treatment of the poisoned person differs according to the type of *argia* that bit him or her" (de Martino, 1966, p. 214–215).

Tarantism, long regarded as a spectacular form of therapy, has been variously interpreted. Some scholars see it "as simply one element in a vast system of symbolic representations one might call astrological in nature"; others see it "as a form of exorcism function-ing within the psychoanalytic logic of a religion based on remorse." Both perspectives "also associate tarantism as a religious phenome-non with possession cults as a whole, but they do so with what one might term repugnance" (Rouget, 1986, p. 159).

Schneider (1948) sees a system of mystical correspondence be-tween nature and human, between the elements, astrological signs, the seasons, and sounds as the cause of the spider dance, which functions "as a form of therapy acting both on the level of accidental reality (that of the illness produced by the spider's bite) and on the level of permanent reality (that of the struggle between life and death, summer and winter, stillness and movement, re-newal and decay). Within the overall configuration of these mystic correspondences, musical sounds, musical instruments, and dance steps occupy a well-defined position. It is by virtue of this position, and of the power it confers upon them, that music and dance en-sure the triumph of recovery, which should simply be seen as an example of the victory of life" (Rouget, 1986, p. 159). Within this theory, the real and the symbolic closely intertwine. Rouget's cri-tique is that the symbolic system Schneider described has never ac-tually been observed and nothing proves that the elements that make it up have ever constituted a whole.

Thirteen years after Schneider's work appeared, de Martino (1961, translated in French, 1966) came to a totally different inter-pretation based on team fieldwork conducted in Salento in 1959. He considers tarantism as a "minor religious form" of exorcism whose origins are likely to be found in the "orgiastic and initiatory cults of classical antiquity." He thinks the actual spider poisoning that the Middle Age Christian armies experienced during the Cru-sade catalyzed the birth of the tarantula symbol. The activities sur-rounding it became an institution which functioned on a "mythico-ritual horizon of recapture and reintegration in relation to critical moments of human existence, with a marked preference for the cri-sis of puberty, the theme of the forbidden eros, and the conflicts of adolescence, within the framework of a peasant lifestyle" (de Martino, 1966, p. 304).

One of the dance figures is an imitation of the spider's movements. With the tarantulee's back to the ground, body arched, movement takes place on all fours. A 17th-century account says that some tarantulees let themselves hang outdoors from trees by ropes or indoors from a rope fixed to a ceiling. More than mere imitation, de Martino interprets this figure as symbolic of the swing of hanged virgins and Phaedra's hanging and thus a sign of frustrated, unhappy, or thwarted female passions. It is also symbolic, he says, of being rocked in a mother's arms and then being temporarily abandoned.

Rouget, however, argues that this best-known example of trance in all of Europe "turns out to be nothing more than a particular form of possession." The essential thing is not exactly what the dancers are trying to rid themselves of but rather how they do it. The dance is placed under the sign of Saint Paul, whose chapel serves as a "theater" for the tarantulees' public meetings. The spider seems to be constantly interchangeable with Saint Paul; the female tarantulees dress as "brides of Saint Paul" and even today sing: "Say where the tarantula stung you / Underneath the hem of my skirt / . . . Oh my Saint Paul of the tarantulas / Who stings all the girls / And makes them saints" (de Martino, 1966, p. 240).

Tarantism, as in other forms of possession, involves entrancement during which the dancer indulges in extravagant behavior, including movement like a spider. Healing from the tarantula bite is the manifest function of tarantism. This, however, provided a providential alibi, for the Church of Rome could never tolerate the existence of an overt possession cult. Women who give themselves up to possession practices in tarantism, however, were not sinners but "unfortunate victims of the spider." Music and dance mechanically expel the venom.

"Possession should be understood as a form of therapy of adversity, bringing into play an institutionalized hysteria or, if one prefers, a socialization of hysteria. Music and dance are precisely the principal means of socializing or institutionalizing this hysteria, by providing it with stereotyped forms of trance, forms that of course depend upon the set of representations constituting the particular system of a given cult. In tarantism, the tarantula (music and dance) does not have the function of curing the tarantulee of her hysteria, but on the contrary, provides her with a means of behaving like an hysteric in public, in accordance with a model recognized by all, thereby freeing her from inner misfortune. How? By providing her with a means of 'coming out of herself' and of communicating with the world, with society, with herself. . . . it must . . . be viewed as a response to a need for communication" (Rouget, 1986, p. 164–65).

There is ambiguity in tarantism, for although the bite is most frequently imaginary, it can sometimes be real. In the latter instance the toxicity causes pain, difficulty in standing, muscular rigidity, sometimes sexual arousal, and a sensation of burning and tingling in the soles of the feet. Besieged by depression, anxiety, and a sense of impending death, the patient then becomes agitated and hallucinatory. "The tingling sensation in the feet and the 'intermittent trembling that occurs principally in the lower limbs (sometimes displaying a convulsive aspect)' obviously constitute, in addition, an invitation to dance" (ibid.).

Within tarantism, "the symbolic and the real, the signifier and the signified, the manifest and the latent, the anecdote and the hidden meaning, the pretext and the profound motivation . . . coincide perfectly. We should not forget, however, that although the purpose is sometimes to chase out the venom and always to expel what it symbolizes, the intention is not to chase out the spider, but, on the contrary, to identify oneself to it, which is done a great deal by imitating it in a variety of different ways" (ibid.).

Irrespective of the different interpretations, we can conclude that tarantism is sometimes a means to deal with stresses of life transitions and conflicts about sexuality, although the initial catalyst was the physical stress of spider venom. The action of tarantism certainly calls attention to the individual who intentionally or otherwise may try to resist, reduce or escape the stresses of life's trials and tribulations. In the ritual, there is the psychological support of the musicians and observers who receive messages of adversity as well as empathize with the physical behavior of catharsis, release, or escape through vigorous movement. When a person is poisoned, the dancing may induce stress that detracts from the stress of the venom.

A literary example of the tarantism phenomenon is Ibsen's *A Doll's House*. Thomas F. Johnston reminded me that the husband forces his unwilling wife to dance it before assembled guests. She eventually asserts her independence.

Black Death

Medieval Europe, an economically harsh and morally complex world, was fought over by God and the devil in a largely preliterate society dominated by the Christian church. Terror of death and anxieties about the repressiveness of state feudalism provoked the compulsion to dance. Dances were a means to cope with the stresses of the day, especially the high mortality rate and short life span. The dances of death visualized an eerie contrast between the youthful vigor of dancing and the eternal stillness of death. Dancing was part of a convivial attempt to deny the finality of death. Emphasizing the terrors of death, the dance was also an attempt to frighten sinners into repentance. Performers would beckon people to the hereafter in response to the epidemic Black Death (1347–73), a bubonic plague in Italy, Spain, France, Germany, and England. Evolving with the skeletal figure seen as our future self, the dance not only mocked the pretenses of the rich who abused their positions on earth, but also pointed to a vision of social equality. The death figure dances convulsively, lording it over mortals who are sent a somber message.

After the harvest in certain years, hallucination, a sense of suffocation and burning, and clonic cramp symptoms of bread and grain ergot (a rye fungus) poisoning, called St. Anthony's Fire, led some of the sickly victims to move involuntarily in dance-like movements. The dancing victims were believed to be possessed by invading demons. Other victims sought relief from pain through ecstatic dancing that matched the convulsive movements of St. John's and St. Vitus's dances, considered of curative value and likely to ward off death. Backman (1952), who identified the association between the symptoms and alkaloid poisoning from ergot, concluded that dancing would indeed provide a symptomatic relief for the victims until the poison had worked its way through their systems. However, the mania for dance was more widespread than the poisoning. Dancing appears to have served key cathartic, working through, and other stress management functions.

Dancing was part of wakes for the dead and the rebirth of the soul to everlasting life. At the graves of family, friends, and martyrs, dancing comforted the dead and encouraged resurrection in addition to protecting them from the dead as demons.

Ketjak

The Balinese *ketjak* (called the Monkey Dance although about humans and only incidentally animals) was a traditional religious performance used during stressful times of peril and pestilence. Ketjak refers to the sounds voiced by a male chorus (in lieu of an orchestra) that accompanies several kinds of dances intended both to stimulate trance states in individuals and to promote purification (*sangyang*) of a village. McKean (1979) witnessed ceremonies that started in December and were performed nightly for four months and then every fifth night for another month. A local priest first prepared offerings and incense. The spirits then incarnated themselves in two young girls about 14 years old. Bodily recipients of *dedari*, meaning heavenly nymphs, they would dance Sangyang Dedari, a dance believed to exorcise evil and bring a blessing. They danced well into the night before emerging from the trance. During this dancing the *ketjak* itself began and lasted for several hours.

From purity to pollution? McKean asks. Since the recent contact with the West, the dance has also become a popular tourist attraction and the sacred and profane coexist. For economic gain, Balinese now perform in tourist hotels. This performance, however, is different in its condensation, selective sharing, and meaning for the participants. Limited to an hour, much that one observes in the traditional ceremony is consequently omitted. Yet, the Balinese retain their religious obligations that follow from devotion to a hierarchy of gods, demons, spirits, and wraiths, which they acknowledge to have power or control over their lives. Moreover, there seems to remain an "intuitive meaning," a "peculiar way of seeing" in the *ketjak* that is not vitiated by the commercial enterprise of tourist entertainment.

Shakers

Dance in its kaleidoscopic variety is sometimes a means to deal with stresses of the sexual drive: the cathartic energy or orgasm of dance simulates and sublimates sexual consummation. A remarkable example is found among the United Society of Believers in Christ's Second Appearing, commonly called the Shakers because of their dramatic practice of vigorous dancing to crush sexual desire and dispel sin. This behavior was related to their belief that the day of judgment was imminent. About 6,000 members in nineteen communities at its peak in the United States, the group said salvation would come through confessing and forsaking fleshly practices. Sexual conduct became a benchmark of an individual's morality and the basis for reward or punishment in the next life. If lust were conquered, other problems would solve themselves.

Ann Lee (1736–84), a founder of this utopian, millenary society, had experiences that played a central role in shaping Shaker theology and practice (Kern, 1981). Lee had deep feelings of guilt and shame about her strong sex drive, a sense of impurity concerning the fleshly cohabitation of the sexes, and a prurient interest in the sex lives of others. Her turbulent marriage led to eight bitter and harrowingly difficult pregnancies. Lee's offspring were stillborn or died in early childhood, only one living to six years. Sexual coition had caused her suffering. During one of her periods of imprisonment (the Shakers were frequently persecuted), she received a revelation of Adam and Eve's first "carnal act," which she interpreted as the source of human depravity. She then promulgated a revulsion toward sexuality.

Lee was concerned with the plight of women in marriage, likened to servitude, prostitution, and rape, and the risks of pregnancy and parturition. Women's bodies were maimed through primitive knowledge of bodily functions (Shorter, 1982). The Shakers thus saw woman as a victim abused by irresponsible men for their selfish pleasure.

Choosing celibacy, Lee became a universal mother and sublimated her sex drives in a spiritualization. "She called herself, and was considered by her followers, the 'Second Appearing of Christ'. . . . As a female Christ she stood in the place of spiritual mate to the male Christ. She is reputed to have told the Elders on one occasion that Christ 'is my Lord and Lover' (a spiritual lover impregnating her with the lives of regenerated souls)" (Kern, 1981, p. 74). A female image of God did empower women in the Shaker community. Their social organization was based on the equality of the sexes and emphasized group rather than individual pursuits.

Notwithstanding Shaker attitudes toward transcending the body through sheer willpower, the first adherents were seized by an involuntary and repressed passion. It led them to run about a meeting room, jump, hop, tremble, whirl, reel in a spontaneous manner, and "wrestle with the Devil" to shake off "the flesh" and doubts, loosen sins and faults, induce humility, and purge the body of lust in order to purify the spirit. Toward repentance they turned away from preoccupation with self to shake off in febrile performance called "laboring" their bondage to a troubled past. The attempt to escape the body while being riveted to it permitted concentration on new feelings and intent. In this working through, individualistic impulsive and ecstatic abandon eventually evolved into ordered, well-rehearsed, drill-like group movement patterns over the 200 years of the sect's existence. Shaking the hand palm downward discarded the carnal, turning palms upward petitioned eternal life. The square, circle, line or march, and endless change comprised the spatial design. Herein male and female often came in proximity to each other, yet they never touched. The shaking-off-sin movement sequence parallels the sexual experience of energy build-up to climax and then relaxation. Both sexes dancing conveyed images of a process of the pursuit of purity and denial of sexuality (Kern, 1981, p. 100; Andrews, 1940, pp. 144–45).

For the Shakers who believed in the dualism of spirit versus body, dancing appears to be a canalization of feeling in the context of men and women living together in celibacy, austerity, humility, and hard manual labor. Dancing afforded an outlet for energies restrained by Shaker regimentation, and a sanctioned emotional release from the enforced separation of the sexes. Men and women were apart except for the worship service, of which dance was a central part, and during the rare "union" or visiting meetings.

Commentary

Tarantism, the dances of death, *ketjak*, and Shakerism encompass religious world views about physical phenomena. The dances were ways of coping with a host of stresses: puberty crises, sexual frustration, spider bites, plagues, ergot poisoning, economic and political exploitation, and lack of attention. Both autogenic and directive styles of dealing with stress were used. The participants' dancing was psychologically and physically cathartic and provided avenues for altered states of consciousness. For the most part, the functions of the dances were not explicitly articulated. The Shakers, however, in their extreme view of sexuality, were clear about the movement shaking off sin, sublimating sexual passion in a sanctioned release.

Use of dance to manage anxiety and fear, involved supportive social networks, symbolic enactments of problems and desired actions, and pretexts for behavior that would not otherwise be acceptable or possible.

Chapter 5
Coming to Terms with Stressful Life Crises

Marriage, Life, and Death in Ubakala Igbo Dance-Plays

Although Nigeria's Ubakala dance-plays can be taken as representative of Africa, bear in mind that Africa has about 2,000 different language groups, and probably that many different dance pattern constellations. Variety does exist (Hanna, 1986a).

Ubakala Igbo dance-plays are conceived, produced, performed, and responded to in terms of an interweaving of the intrinsic characteristics of the dance-play genre and the extrinsic characteristics of Ubakala culture and society. An examination of this interweaving, on the basis of my field experience (1976, 1987d), showed the dance-plays to be the expression of emotion or its symbolization, as well as the expression of ideas. As such, the dance-play appears to be a psychotherapeutic vehicle for the diagnosis, prevention, and treatment of stress-related personal and social disorder. It serves as catharsis, anticipatory psychic management, and paradox mediation (discussed in Chapter 6).

The dance-play serves to prevent illness as a result of stress. A communicative modality, the dance-play engages an individual with potentially stressful concerns in a communal activity with persons close to him or her (see Frank, 1973, p. 318, on family and community therapy for mental illness). Similarly, in the dance-play the Ubakala present stressful grievances for conflict resolution. Because some of the Ubakala values are contradictory and the pursuit of one to the exclusion of the other creates a paradox, the dance-play becomes diagnostic through its presentation of the issues and mediatory through its catalyst of remedial action.

A few basic contextual facts are relevant to understanding the functioning of the dance-play in helping people with potentially stressful life crises. The Ubakala are one of about 200 formerly politically autonomous Igbo groups in Nigeria. In terms of social organization, the Ubakala are patrilineal and patrilocal, that is, descent is traced on the father's side, and a married couple and their children live with the father's family. There is a sexually based division of agricultural labor, in part biologically determined on the basis of reproductive and physical strength capabilities. Reincarnation and ancestor honor are key tenets in the traditional polytheistic religion which persists to some degree even among converted Christians. They may add Jesus to the pantheon.

The function of dance-plays (*nkwa*) among the Ubakala appears to approximate the human potential or self-actualization model of dance therapy and the preventive medicine, or wellness, model rather than the medical model. Ubakala dance-plays help to maintain cultural patterns and provide stability for individuals, that is, norms for social life are presented in the performances. The dance-play is a method of indoctrination about the individual's role, sense of self-worth, and group support. Through the *nkwa*, individuals have a medium to assist them in achieving their fullest potential, to adapt to the social environment, and to change distasteful aspects of the social milieu. The dance-play reflects, influences, and is part of many other aspects of the society and culture in which it is embedded. Dance may be viewed as a language of command and control, that is, a vehicle of power—defined as the ability to influence others' predispositions, feelings, attitudes, beliefs, and actions.

Specific mechanisms of dance-play "group therapy" focus on preventing stress by engaging in "anticipatory psychic management" of life crises (Hanna and Hanna, 1968) and "alternative catharsis."

(1) A method of socialization, *anticipatory psychic management* prepares an individual for a threatening experience by rehearsing it until its potential destructive emotional impact is reduced to

manageable proportions. "Systematic desensitization" (Wolpe, 1958) is the equivalent terminology used in behavior modification. "Every fresh repetition," wrote Freud, "seems to strengthen this mastery for which [the individual] strives (1955, pp. 14–17). The therapeutic efficacy is not in sheer repetition but "active reproduction or recreation and . . . transformation through various mechanisms, characteristic of artistic production" (Bychowski, 1951, p. 393).

Usually, repetition in order to manage or assimilate a situation or feeling relates to a past traumatic event. However, repetition can also help manage anticipated future events. Among the Ubakala, anticipatory psychic management appears to be most commonly associated with the tensions of adulthood, for example, getting married, giving birth, and coping with death. Typical of anticipating womanhood is the *Nkwa Edere* (young girls' shimmy dance-play). In several of the specific dances, the movement refers to anxieties and emotional occasions in the life of an adult woman, namely, heterosexual relations, becoming a wife and leaving one's natal home, being fertile, and giving birth. Young girls within the age of puberty (11 to 16 years old) focus on the hazards they will most likely face as they pass into adulthood.

The dance *Ogbede Turuime* ("pregnant child") refers to a small girl's fear that when she marries she may be infertile and when she becomes pregnant might not deliver successfully. The dance's foci, the anxieties of becoming fertile and of childbirth (a dangerous process without modern medical treatment, in which tragedy may occur for seemingly inexplicable reasons), have even broader anticipatory relevance: the transition from childhood to adulthood. This transition is more traumatic for a girl than for a boy because for her, marriage means leaving the familiar home environment to live among strangers—her husband and his kin (among whom she is not fully accepted as a family member)—and at the same time adjusting to her new roles of wife and mother. "Being a wife . . . is no easy matter" (Okonkwo, 1971, p. 149). At the separation of a bride from her ancestral lineage, elderly women console the girl and her mother by reminding them that what is involved is a journey and not death. In fact, young brides are known to run away to their birthplace from home sickness.

In *Nkwa Edere*, the shoulders shimmy in many of the dance movements as the pelvis shifts from side to side. Breast development and other pubescent body changes are thus highlighted. Girls dance on their knees in a one-two-three-hold Conga pattern in one of the movement variations; the torso is forward-inclined as if entreating the beneficence of the fruit-giving earth deity for human fertility.

Aspects of both the *Nkwa Uko* (dance-play for the death of an aged woman) and the *Nkwa Ese* (dance-play for the death of an aged man) can be interpreted as anticipatory psychic management because they familiarize participants with the rituals accompanying death, reminding them of the coming of their own deaths and their opportunity to eventually achieve ancestor status (cf. Keleman, 1975). The *Nkwa Uko* dance entitled "The Deceased are Blessed" suggests this.

These dance-plays for the deceased appear to release the living from the stresses imposed by a death in a way that is minimally disruptive, to give the living an opportunity to anticipate and thus better manage their lives in regard to their own demise, and to communicate the clan's beliefs about life and death.

The death of a friend or relative creates problems of psychological stress for the living as mentioned earlier. Second burials (rituals to assist the buried deceased in her or his journey to the ancestor world) and other mourning ceremonies constitute institutionalized means of working through the problems gradually. If all affect were discharged at once, the twofold result could be overwhelming individual stress and group disruption. The communal solidarity experienced in the *nkwa* and the physical expenditure of tension in its performance help to improve group morale and dissipate anxiety; it is a psychological support for members of the bereaved family, for whom death has disturbed existing social and ritual relationships and of whom adjustment is demanded. Thus the dance-plays appear to provide a useful vehicle for tension release and prevention of stress.

Despite the universality of death, its rationalization, and the Ubakala belief that ancestors are the continuation of a lineage's living representatives, considerable anxiety about death still exists (see Uchendu, 1965, p. 12). Umunna (1968, p. 178) tells us that the first reactions to death for the Igbo are disgust, annoyance, pain, and a sense of loss, for death is indiscriminate in killing good and wicked alike. The Ottenbergs write: "This anxiety is often well hidden in formalized ways of talking about illness, or in cure-seeking rituals . . . every blessing, be it of the ancestors in the serving of palm wine, be that a sacrifice, contains the statement, 'Let there be long life'" (1964, p. 31).

In the *Nkwa Ese* dance-play for a deceased man, dancing out the apparent anger in response to death is a form of symbolic concretization involving the transformation of a wish, thought, or mood into a mock interpersonal encounter. It externally fixed and codifies feelings that have been repressed or concealed.

Through machete and stick brandishing advances and retreats, the male dancers in the *Nkwa Ese* vigorously portray as warrior-like the deeds, exploits, and prowess of the deceased or his ancestors in order to bestow praise and honor upon him and his descendants. In the *Nkwa Uko*, the women dance in much the same way as they do for the celebration of a birth of a child. However, physical contact occurs occasionally when two women, each with an arm around the other's waist, dance together at the center of the circle, perhaps as a sign of condolence.

In a society whose religious beliefs include reincarnation, participating in a ceremony concerning the death of another may give individuals an opportunity to cope more effectively with the stresses associated with the coming of their own deaths. This coping mechanism is most evident when the ceremony emphasizes generational continuity and praises the dead.

(2) *Catharsis*, another dance-play group therapy mechanism to prevent stress, is experienced through enervating movements, deviant movement patterns, and/or transgressive criticism. The *enervating movements* of Ubakala girls' and women's dance-plays appear to provide catharsis for females' empathic fears about the uncertainties of a successful birth, sanctions for failure, and pain

related to marriage and childbirth. Similarly the dance-plays for the deceased provide outlets for emotional stress that accompanies the loss of a loved one and fear of the deceased's spirit.

A newborn child represents the triumph over the odds of infant mortality. Large families are necessary for agricultural work; protection; security in old age; and a manpower reservoir capable of replacing the victims of infant mortality, war, and disease—for perpetuation of the group. Having offspring marks success in life. Children are required to perform the dance-play to ensure the deceased's journey to the world of the ancestors, from which rebirth occurs as a grandchild or other incarnation. Death is seen as merely the terminus of one phase of time and space. "For a person to die without children to perform funeral rituals for him is a tragedy. Implicitly it means, of course, that he is soon likely to be forgotten, for who will sacrifice to him as an ancestor?" (Ottenbergs, 1964, p. 31). Who will "offer . . . the daily prayers, libations of wine, and sacrifices of kola nuts or pieces of food?" (Ilogu, 1965, p. 338). Having many surviving children brings a parent prestige and marks success in life. Indeed, an Ubakala woman's marriage and personal status depends on this.

Yet, childbirth has its hazards, as we have noted. The dance-play performed to rejoice for the birth of a child appears to provide a safety-valve mechanism for the release of women's emphathic delivery tension, pain, and anxiety about infant mortality—emotions that might otherwise be directed toward relatively dysfunctional activities. In deference to the pregnant women participating, the dance tempo is slow and the movement texture sustained; however, anxiety may be reduced through continuous motion, full-throated song, and explosive yells and ululations. Perhaps as compensation for being considered the inferior sex in a male-dominated society, this vivid dance-play, which proclaims the great achievement of women, is a means of female self-assertion.

Dance is often restorative in allowing an individual to reassert the impulsive after the strain of adapting and the weariness of conforming. *Deviant movement patterns*, a form of catharsis, occur in the *Nkwa Edere* waltz dance. In pairs, the girls embrace and caress each other as they dance. The embracing European ballroom dance position is a parody of male-female behavior which is not traditionally approved (but occurs in the urban areas). Public physical contact between men and women is not seen in Ubakala villages. Safier writes: "Convention dictates which postures, stance, carriage or gait we assume in this or that area of life. Dance is perceived as an escape from this restraint although dance brings with it its own bondage: in the stylization of movements. At least, dance movements are different from the movements of routine living. Thus dance encourages relaxation both in reality and in illusion" (1953, p. 242).

Transgressive criticism through the dance-play, which serves as a legitimate vehicle for otherwise prohibited or inappropriate social commentary and criticism, joking, or aggression, may be cathartic. Nwoga argues that the salutary function of satire (socialization to proper attitudes and behavior) is incidental to the "idea of punishment through words. It is anger with a person or a group, rather than the sense of offended morality which is the principal urge" (1971, p. 34).

Samburu Role Transition and Dance

Another case of catharsis and coming to terms with crises in the life cycle comes from northern Kenya. Here, the Samburu dances are both markers and outlets for stresses related to passage from one phase of the life cycle to another. Boys eagerly look forward to initiation into warriorhood, the privileges of which, including close association with girls, are jealously guarded by the existing *moran*, or warrior, age-set. The age-set of *moran* retires to elderhood at about 30 years of age, marrying and settling down when the next age-set, about 14 years younger, takes over. The assertiveness of the boys' circumcision dance is an expression of their restlessness and anticipation of circumcision. There is an implicit element of coercion in the boys uniting in dance to demand circumcision because it legitimates them as a new set of future warriors.

The dances of the *moran*, young warriors prohibited from marrying in an order imposed by the elders, according to Spencer's evaluation of the evidence, seem to point convincingly towards a temporary release of the tension that is built up among young people associated with their restricted position in society. The Samburu's flexible nomadic existence makes a monogamous family too small to be economically viable as an independent house unit. Consequently, the Samburu have developed a social organization with polygyny, a delayed age of marriage for men, and leadership by mature adult men who monopolize formal power and nubile women. In the interim a *moran* can have a young adolescent mistress within his clan although he cannot marry her. Older women are married and involved in homemaking activities.

There is a concerted force manifest in a suppressed sector of Samburu society. "The *moran* and girls [who join the *moran* in special dances] do not merely release tension, but they also develop a camaraderie, united through the dance in a token protest against the regime under which they are placed" (Spencer, 1985, p. 155). The dancing provides a gauge of sentiment that the elders cannot ignore when they see the dance reigning supreme with its alternative undomesticated order.

In preparation for a dance, the *moran* carefully adorn themselves with their loin cloths and glistening red ochre around their faces and shoulders. They try to outdo each other in self-display and boasting in the dance. At first the *moran* usually dance *nbarinkoi*. In a tight chanting group they rhythmically move forward together, "twice raising their heels, bending their knees, thrusting their heads forwards and exhaling audibly—in fact not unlike bulls—and then straightening themselves and lifting their spears on the third beat." At times a *moran* individually may hop away from the group and then return.

The *nkokorri* dancing has provocative thrusting movements with assertive bull-like grunting followed by jumping movement as the dancers rise and fall in unison. Shivering movement climaxes the dance. A display of the urge to fight and of manliness, as well as an act that makes a man irresistible in battle, the shivering accompanies a "tightness gripping their chests, inducing a sense of breathless suffocation as they sink into unconsciousness and achieve relaxation" (pp. 147–148). The girls, who have also carefully adorned themselves for the occasion of the dance, look on. After these two male dances of display, the girls as a group join in the dance. Taunting the youths to engage in cattle rustling, the girls partake in vicarious rebelliousness.

"The principal weapon of the elders is their control over the marriages of their daughters, which override the more transient claims of the *moran* over these girls. It is the elders who decide when each bond between lovers should terminate by marrying the girl off to some other clan, where she will start a new life in a position of complete subservience. Thus each wedding is a sharp reminder for all *moran* and girls of the elders' power to interfere in their affairs, and significantly this is the principal occasion at which *moran* are popularly expected to express their protest in a display of anger through dancing" (pp. 144–45). Yet, the dance is one of the opposed forces of assertiveness and constraint. Very angry *moran* may "break down in an insensible fit of convulsive shaking" (p. 147) in response to the paradoxical stress. At successful dances, as many as five or more *moran* will break down in this way, following each other in relatively quick succession. "And then after the shaking subsides and they regain their composure, they return to the dance apparently cured of their bout of anger as they merge almost passively into the main body of dancers.

Married men do not dance. However, married women have their dances for fertility. These dances provide a measure of temporary escape from domestic chores and dominance by the males.

Lugbara Dances for Death and Life's Uncertainty

Through their dancing, the Lugbara of Uganda convey messages about their desire for a stable society that in fact never is; the social and cosmic relations in which they are involved are always uncertain and beyond their comprehension. The dance is one means by which they try "to comprehend and so control or resolve situations of structural ambiguity" (Middleton, 1985, p. 166).

Anticipatory psychic management is operative in dances related to death. The Lugbara, like the Ubakala, mark the process of change from living to dead in rites of transition. "At death the constituent elements of the person separate and move from the social sphere to those beyond it. The soul goes to Divinity in the sky, the spirit to the wilderness. . . .the soul is later redomesticated by diviners and the spirit remains in the bushland. During this process the social status of the deceased is uncertain, beyond contact by the living, who cannot enter into any direct relationship with him or her: after the establishment of a shrine they may do so again" (p. 167).

Integral to Lugbara mortuary rites are two dances. Wailing dances, *ongo* or *auwu-ongo*, take place soon after a death, sometimes even prior to the actual burial. They show respect to the deceased, who would otherwise be insulted and possibly send sickness or nightmares to his living kin or appear to them as a specter. Playing dances (*abi* or *avico-ongo*) are performed a year after a death. The lineage members of the deceased dance and wail, whereas the affines (those related by marriage) "play" to create and show joy that disrupted lineage and kinship ties have been reaffirmed. The order of dancing, with each group praising the prowess of its own lineage segments and attacking the others, expresses the constellation of lineage ties that has been disrupted by death. The death dance for an important man may attract well over a hundred people, some of whom become drunk and aggressive.

A special feature of the dance is a trancelike condition after a longer period of performance and drinking on a relatively empty stomach. This may link the dancers to the soul and other elements of the deceased in a form of individuality, a dramatic retreat from customary relations with others within the lineage group.

The dance participants are primarily men who dance as a group. In two lines set within a circle of onlookers, the men leap up and down in inward concentration with legs straight and together, arms either stretched out above their head or holding weapons, symbols of masculinity. Women, by contrast, dance individually or as groups of sisters; they hop loosely and hold their arms out in front of them at shoulder level, bent at the elbow in a supple waving gesture.

There are women's dances that bear certain resemblance to death dances in that they are performed when there is uncertainty. Women dance *nyambi* as an intervention for anxiety immediately after an exceptionally productive harvest or after one delayed due to excessive rain and at the end of a long dry season. During these disorderly, irregular times, intergroup quarreling and fighting over scarce resources is common. The women dance to the raingrove, where the rainmaker awaits them and then performs rites to reset the orderly passing of time and repair social relations. Seemingly a mirror reflection of the death dance in which men dance in lines of patrilineal kin, women of the subclan dance together irrespective of lineage and affinal affiliations. (See earlier discussion of the Gogo.)

Dance and Transformation: Death/Disorder to Life/Order

Stress management occurs in dance rituals of transformation. At life crises, these performances permit individuals to anticipate future crises as well as accept them in a positive vein through catharsis. In Tanzania the Nyakyusa's funeral dance begins with a passionate expression of anger and grief and gradually becomes a fertility dance. In this way dancing mediates the passionate and quarrelsome emotions felt over a death and the acceptance of it, the uncontrolled and controlled (Wilson, 1954).

Among the Dogon of Mali, death creates a special kind of disorder. Yet through the dance, humans metaphorically restore order to the disordered world in a like-equals-reality conception. Symbolically spatializing a world they have not seen, the Dogon illustrate the representation of heaven on earth, their cosmic image conventionally reflected in arranging villages by pairs, one representing heaven, the other earth, their fields cleared spirally as the world is believed to have been created. So, too, at the time of death, the mask dance occurs to help the community deal with the psychic distress and spiritual fear of the dead. Order exists in the dancing with its specific symbolism and patterns in the spheres of sociocultural event, total human body (conceived of as an image of the cosmos) in action, organic and discursive performance, specific movements, and other communication, particularly costume (Griaule, 1965).

Commentary

We have seen how the dance medium is a vehicle through which people come to terms with hallmarks of life—birth, death, and uncertainty. The rituals, through anticipation, catharsis, group protest, altered states of consciousness, and symbolic enactment, allow people resist stress, reduce it when it occurs, or temporarily escape it. The stress intervention style is autogenic, although social and cultural tradition is directive in providing expectations for the dance performance.

Chapter 6
Resolving Conflict and Ameliorating Stress

This chapter includes two cases of secular social/ethnic dance that illustrate how dance is a communicative medium to move people to consider ideas and actions in order to resolve a stressful situation. The reports derive from my field work in Africa in the 1960s and in the United States in the 1970s. I will discuss the Ubakala use of dance in social drama in Nigeria and Afro-American play with dance in a Dallas school. Herein we have problems of females and blacks, groups that have their unique stressors.

Relevant to these cases is the concept of dance as play. Play may be a school or practice, a safe arena for exploring beyond the known or working through problems, an exercise of mental or physical faculties, and an activity of survival value. It is a derivation from life situations of flight, fight, sex, and eating behavior. Schechner points out that play maintains a "regular, crisis-oriented expenditure of kinetic energy" that can be "switched from play-energy into fight-energy." (1973, p. 33)

Ubakala Social Drama

An Ubakala dance-play that illustrates the prevention and reduction of stress when it occurs is the 'outsider" relations' society dance-play. The society originated as an expression of unity by related women who marry into the same village. Their goals are to rejoice in the fact that they have children, to confront jointly the problems of family life, to share economic resources, and to affirm friendships among married women originally from the same village. Living as they do among "strangers" where they have little part in formal political and religious activities, women who hail from the same village seek each other out. This can be seen as their attempt as "outsiders" to counter the bonds of blood and kin that bind their husbands. These women especially use the dance-play to adjust wrongdoings and work through the contradictions of social life.

Paradox mediation, a form of stress prevention and remediation, refers to the resolution of conflicting opposites. Fundamental and sometimes conflicting, Ubakala values move people to social action. An emphasis on individualistic competition and achievement is juxtaposed with the need for cooperation and interdependence (community spirit, group solidarity, and sharing the wealth: personal aggrandizement is not emphasized). The desire for and expectation of change often run counter to the principle of respect for authority, which is largely based on seniority. Innovation generally involves criticism or rejection of what those older than oneself have established. The principle of respect and obedience to leaders is opposed both to the egalitarian distaste for assertive authority, and to the norm of bringing things into the open.

If an individual or group pursues one part of a pair of opposites to the exclusion of the other, this creates an imbalance, dilemma, and social drama. When one value is expressed such that it violates another equally valid value and an individual or group feels threatened and desires to contain, modify, or reverse it, the dance-play mediates between persons and their situations (in much the same way as speech mediates between persons and their situations or a shaman mediates unbalanced forces in a healing ritual). Mediation refers to reconciling action.

The dance-play has the potential to mediate social relations and political situations by encapsulating the issues and phases of social dramas. The four phases of social drama are (1) a breach of the norms of a social group, (2) a mounting crisis, (3) a legal or ritual redressive process, and (4) public and symbolic expression of an irreparable schism or conciliation (Turner, 1974). Accordingly, the dance-play may communicate the breach, foment the crisis, ameliorate the conflict (or at least hold it in suspension so that it is present, viewable, and ponderable), and proclaim the schism or celebrate the reintegration.

Ubakala allow a special kind of license in the dance-play that protects the individual and group from libel. Alternative social arrangements can be played with, exciting programs undermined, and new ones generated. Contrary ways of acting and thinking, perhaps ultimately unworkable or with disastrous consequences, or normative ways with positive impact may be presented. The dance-play is a vehicle for negotiating separate personalities, individual biographies, into a shared entity to transform personal experience and thus create a certain degree of anonymity.

The dance-play has the potential for more than letting off steam or *catharsis*: It can guard against the misuse of power and produce social change without violence. However, dance-play messages are often implicit; and a symbolic system is a weak vehicle of control unless enforcement follows. The dance-play is a *political form of coercion* in a shame-oriented society. Energy (force), the ultimate means of social control, is symbolically represented.

The famous 1929 "women's war" in which the dance-play communication went unheeded illustrates the potential of this women's medium. Repercussions were widespread both on local and intercontinental levels. Contemporary politicians and leaders refer to this notorious episode of feminine protest (Gailey, 1970, provides one of the fullest accounts) as reason for considering women's views. They remember how the women moved the mighty British to alter their colonial administration of eastern Nigeria.

Women's intrusion into the affairs of state and their imposition of sanctions makes them the custodians of the "constitution" (Njaka, 1974, p. 22). Because women marry outside the village group into which they were born, their kin organization cuts across and goes beyond any one level of political structure. The organization is thus potentially powerful in rallying numerous groupings behind any single member.

As a boycott, the women's dance-play is sometimes called "sitting on a man" (Van Allen, 1972; Dorward, 1982). The aggrieved gather at the compound of an offender and dance and sing to detail the problem. Movement presents a dynamic image emphasizing the argument as well as releasing and generating physical and psychological energy and tension. The accompanying song, with its potent ridicule and satire, serves as a vehicle for specific social criticism.

The British colonial government of Nigeria was generally aware of the potential for public disturbance in this cultural expression. Thus its native council was empowered by the 1901 Proclamation, Section 36(3) to regulate "native plays . . . [gatherings] of natives in any public street or market, or in any house, building, or in any compound adjoining a public street or market for the purpose of dancing or playing native music" (City Ordinance 591/2 in Nwabara 1965, pp. 188–89). In some areas licenses and permission from the British District Commissioner were necessary to hold plays.

A *breach* of understanding between women and the colonial government began the first phase of the women's war social drama. In 1928 the British government introduced taxation applicable to men. Late in 1929 women incorrectly believed that this tax was to be extended to them. This misunderstanding signaled the beginning of an example of "sex solidarity and political power which women can exercise when they choose to do so" (Meek, 1937, p. 201).

The women viewed taxation as an infringement upon their economic competitive patterns. In the latter part of the 19th century, women started to amass considerable wealth from the growing trade in palm kernels, a women's crop. Not appreciating the economic and political position of women, the British attempted to focus hitherto diffuse power on colonial government-appointed Nigerian male warrant chiefs. Since women had not become representatives of the colonial government, as Nigerian men had, they did not see the benefits from the imposition of taxes. The women's economic and political grievances coalesced. Women were aggrieved by the European control of market prices and what they considered abusive and extortionist practices of many colonial government-appointed Nigerian warrant chiefs (for example, some obtained wives without paying full bride wealth; others took property improprietously).

In the midst of a depression era, the effects of which hurt women, the spark igniting the conflagration was supplied by a young British assistant district officer in Bende Division. (This was the same division where the district officer, A. L. Weir, deceived the people in 1927 about the purpose of the initial tax census.) Because census registers were incomplete and inaccurate, the administrative officers were supposed to revise the initial counts in their spare time. In October, Captain John Cook (who had taken over from Weir) decided on his own authority to obtain information on the number of men, women, children, and livestock.

The massive protest was incited when the Warrant Chief Okugo, of Oloko Village near the town of Aba, employed a school teacher, Mark Emeruwa, to take charge of the census. Inquiring about the possessions of a local woman Nwanyeruwa, the messenger engaged in argument and physical scuffle with her. She then reported the incident to her village women's meeting.

A mounting *crisis*, as women gathered to discuss what had occurred, marked the second phase of the social drama. The alarmed women sent palm leaves, symbols of warning and distress, to women of neighboring and distant villages summoning them to Okoko to join the protest. Women from far and near, even pregnant women, met in the Okoko square on November 24.

The third stage was the potentially *redressive* process of "sitting on a man" which usually works to resolve conflicts and ward off stress. (The audience-captivating dance-play medium serves as a socially acceptable vehicle to express strong displeasure which in turn has the effect of catalyzing people to act to ameliorate the cause of dissatisfaction.) The irate women trooped to the mission that employed Emeruwa, the chief's messenger, to demonstrate against him. They camped in front of his compound at the Niger Delta Mission and "sat on him"—the man was kept from sleeping and carrying out his usual tasks. They danced and sang outside the Mission compound all night, eating, drinking palm wine, and singing that Nwanyeruwa had been told to count her goals, sheep, and people (Nwabara, 1965, p. 231). A song was quickly improvised to meet the situation. The women sent their message. Yet, no satisfactory response was forthcoming.

The next day, with the problem still unresolved, the social drama reached the *schism* phase. The women became more excited and went to the chief's compound. They besieged Chief Okugo at his house and demanded his cap of office, a symbol of authority. He escaped to seek refuge on the Native Court compound. Captain Cook met over 25,000 women in the market to assure them they were not to be taxed; however, the women insisted that Chief Okugo and Emeruwa be arrested and tried.

Skeptical of government assurances that they were not to be taxed, the women's rampages began to spread. Late in December, the women forced the Umuahia warrant chiefs to surrender their caps. In Aba women sang and danced to no avail about their antipathy toward the chiefs and the court messengers. Then they proceeded to attack and loot the European trading stores and Barclays Bank and to break into the prison and release the prisoners (Perham, 1937, p. 208).

The riots spread, involving about ten thousand women in two provinces. Destruction was directed primarily toward the warrant chiefs and buildings representing this detested authority. Finally, in panic the British authorities called troops and police into the area. The most extreme violence was triggered by a car accident and heated passions. In the town of Opobo in Calabar Province, the police opened fire in one of the worst episodes; 32 women were killed and 31 wounded. (See Nigerian Government Reports, 1930a and 1930b; Perham, 1937, pp. 206–220; Onwuteaka, 1965). News of the slaughter spread and local disturbances persisted well into 1930.

The women's rapid mobilization was possible because of their strong societal organizations and effective communication networks based on concentration in the markets and dispersal along the trade routes. Colonial government reorganizations in 1930–31 followed reports of two commissions of inquiry and anthropological study. The women succeeded in their destruction of the warrant chief system. The cost and stress would have been less had the audience been more attentive initially. Thus the contemporary women's dance-play performance serves as a metaphor for their power (cf. Hanna, 1988c).

Related to the memories or stories of dramatic instances of unheeded dance-plays is the dynamic concept of play which may help to explain the role of the dance-play in conflict management. Play, as mentioned earlier, can maintain a pattern of kinetic energy which can be drawn upon for a crisis situation.

In presenting this case of women's social protest, I have tried to suggest that although Ubakala men dominate the traditional political organization and ritual of the egalitarian society with its pattern of tracing descent through the paternal side and family residence among the husband's kin, the women also have power. They perpetuate the husband's lineage, integrate villages through marriage ties, and mediate imbalances in social life as viewed from the perspective of Ubakala values. Rather than being a "muted" group, the women express their wishes and power in dance-plays. Thus they attempt to resist or reduce stress.

The women can transform the dance-play performances into usually persuasive boycotts called "sitting on a man" and dance and sing their grievances. However, when their dance-play communication goes unheeded both in a usual performance and a boycott, the women can switch from playfully dancing to violently waging war—their ultimate means of enforcing their will. The 1929 women's war was a dramatic extension of the traditional method women used to settle grievances with men who acted badly toward them, and thus prevent or reduce stress. There is no escape but a direct confrontation.

Race Relations in Dallas

The expression through dance of complaints to deal with stressful situations is widespread in Africa. Moreover, the arts as a medium to critique society characterizes performance elsewhere in the world. Therefore it is not surprising to find Afro-American children dancing out their reactions to stressful events and ongoing social exchanges.

Needless to say, slavery and its aftermath have been difficult for blacks in the new world. Even desegregation, intended by public policy-makers to be helpful to blacks, was anxiety-producing. Let me share with you some of my observations from a year-long study of Pacesetter, a school in Dallas, Texas (Hanna, 1982, 1986b, 1987b). At the time, Pacesetter was newly desegregated with a court-ordered 50/50 black/white ratio in each classroom. Located in a black neighborhood, the magnet school, because of a superior program, attracts volunteer whites who are bused.

I probably would have dismissed the black children's spontaneous dancing I observed over a year as merely play, as did the school staff, except for my experience in Africa where I discovered the dance both reflected and influenced people's lives. Individuals danced their ethnic identity in the same way that their dress or military emblems announced who they were. Old and young alike used the medium of dance to comment on contemporary problems and solutions. So, what was going on at Pacesetter when children spontaneously danced?

Anthropologists look at the context of activities they seek to understand. So we do not view children's own dancing in school in isolation from the values and experiences of the communities which feed the schools. We also look to the past to help explain creative behavior that can exist for its own sake or be a defensive and stress-coping reaction.

Historically blacks were forced to live in segregated places and often permitted some self-governance. Then, when whites realized the value of black areas for roads, airports, and white residences, or blacks began living too close, whites pushed the blacks out. Verbal intimidation, water well destruction, home bombings, and rezoning laws encouraged black relocation.

Pacesetter school is located in a black community that was created in the 1950s as a result of firebombing of black homes that were purchased or being built in formerly all-white residential areas—nine unsolved explosions in 1951! At the time there was a housing shortage. The black population in Dallas had increased from about 50,000 in 1940 to about 80,000 in 1950, leaving 8,000 families in need of housing. Through the efforts of civic leaders in the Dallas Citizens Interracial Association, a segregated housing project was undertaken within the city limits so that government regulatory services could be provided. The new community of one-story frame houses had its own shopping center, churches, and school.

Desegregation changed the black control of the school. A five-year U.S. Justice Department effort culminated in 1975 when the presiding judge accepted a plan for whites to be bused voluntarily to Pacesetter. The black community was originally middle class, so school and community leaders thought the values of blacks and whites would be similar. However, when laws passed against seg-regated housing, many middle-income blacks moved into other more affluent neighborhoods.

At Pacesetter, desegregation brought together black and white, neighborhood friendship groups and individual volunteers to be bused to the school who were strangers to each other and the black children, and low-income (mostly black) and middle-income (mostly white) youngsters. The majority of black children had been together since preschool. Like friendship groups else-where, they did not always readily accept strangers, even if the strangers were black.

The black community was not unanimously in favor of desegre-gation. Because black-white proximity in the past led to harass-ment of blacks, there was understandable mistrust and anxiety. Desegregation was stressful because blacks feared mistreatment and embarrassment. The white volunteers to Pacesetter, on the other hand, tended to come from civil rights-oriented families and invite interracial friendships. Yet many black children felt the white volunteers at the court-ordered desegregated magnet school were invading their turf.

Although black children born during the late 1960s and 1970s era of "black power" assertiveness may not have been discrimi-nated against, members of their families were. Thus the children were sensitive to anything that could possibly be interpreted as rac-ism. They were wary of the whites who "took over their school." It had a totally black faculty during segregation. However, with de-segregation there were only two black teachers out of a total of 40, one black assistant teacher out of 20 (though there were both black and white co-principals and counselors).

An assumption of desegregation is that low-income blacks will want to emulate middle-class whites and pick up their academic achievement patterns. However, in Pacesetter (as in schools throughout the country), two grade levels behind middle-class whites and blacks in academic achievement, the majority of low-income black children did not highly value academic achievement and do what is required to earn high marks. Indeed, some deval-ued and belittled the ethics and activities of formal school and tried to disrupt the efforts of those who attempted to succeed.

Because of limited employment opportunities for blacks, educa-tion did not have the same positive pay-off as it did for whites. And in the face of limited opportunity, there has not been strong family and community support for black children's academic success.

In spite of the low esteem for academic success some black chil-dren have, they are still sensitive to public criticism of their inade-quate school work. This leads them to seek arenas in which they can dominate and gain recognition. If one has few material posses-sions and little power in the adult world, as is the case with op-pressed minorities and children, the body and its use become especially important. Dance and football were arenas black young-sters selected for excelling at Pacesetter.

Because children learn that what they say with words can get them into trouble, they often use body language to express their frustrations, anxiety, and what is considered inappropriate. Dance appears to be a type of communication that protects the young-sters' defiant thoughts and actions from the negative sanctions of the teacher or other school authority. Purposefully ambiguous, the sender of the message reserves the prerogative to insist on a harm-less interpretation rather than a provocative one.

Let us spotlight three illustrations that suggest how black girls used the dance to deal with the stresses of having white teachers and class-mates in a society with a history of racial discrimination.

Illustration 1. One day during an unusual 40-minute second grade classroom period before the teacher had established control, several black children yelled out remarks; walked about the room; played with furniture pretending it was gymnastic, musical, or military equipment; and pushed, pulled, or hit others. A black boy tried to cut a white girl's blond hair. A black girl kept talking loudly. In response to the white teacher's question, "Would you like to go out? the youngster got up from her chair and walked into the aisle where she stood, feet apart and knees bent. She brought her knees together and apart four times while crossing her hands together and apart in unison with the knees in a Charleston step. Then she scurried back to her assigned seat and sat down. Moments later she skipped to the door, opened it, picked up a book that was lying outside, and ran back to her place. Then she stood upon the chair seat and performed what in ballet is called an "arabesque." Standing on the ball of one foot, she lifted the other leg backward as high as she could, one arm held diagonally up and forward, the other diagonally down. From this position she laughingly lost her balance and fell to the floor. The teacher picked her up and carried her out of the classroom. During the girls' performance, her peers gave her their undivided attention.

The girl's dance movements can be construed as dramatically defying the white teacher by acting inappropriately during a formal lesson. Breaking the rules of both the white-dominated school and of traditional ballet style, the child mocked the teacher. Mockery, of course, is a way to deal with stress. The girl left her assigned seat and walked into the aisle to perform a Charleston movement—part of the repertoire of several black African groups and part of her Afro-American ethnic identity. Then, again, out of the appropriate time and place, she performed an arabesque movement—part of the elitist, white ethnic ballet tradition. To add a further incongruity, the child performed a dance movement—usually danced on a stage floor—on the seat of a classroom chair. Feet were placed where the buttocks are supposed to be. Breaking these rules, the child sassed the teacher in a display of subordination. Her deliberately clumsy fall, performing a movement that traditionally requires the dancer to assume a basic pose and then change the body support on one leg with elegant and graceful body control, was more than mere clown-like action.

The performance suggests once again the historical pattern of blacks parodying white behavior (Hansen, 1967; Levine, 1977). Note that radio and television coverage of Arthur Mitchell in Dallas made common knowledge the history of ballet as a European tradition and formerly studied, performed, and viewed by whites. News commentators repeatedly said that until Mitchell founded the Dance Theatre of Harlem, there were few black ballet dancers. Mitchell came to Dallas periodically to teach, and Pacesetter offered extracurricular ballet classes. In this way blacks learned the ballet rules well enough not only to execute them but to break them.

The child appeared to engage in sympathetic magic in the sense of symbolically enacting, through body motion, wished-for behavior in another realm. When she collapsed her arabesque pose in lieu of concluding it with the traditional ballet aplomb, she seemed to symbolize or, with the compelling power of metaphor, to effect the white teacher's complete downfall from authority.

Illustration 2. At least once a week I saw one to six black children at a time spontaneously dance a few steps in short sequences in a variety of situations both inside and outside the classroom in ways that did not disrupt formal teaching and learning. For example, as a second grade class was being dismissed, one black boy exited performing a Charleston step three times. This was the same step the black girl performed in the first illustration. After the first boy exited, a second black boy followed performing the same movement phrase. The sequence occurred repeatedly until six black boys had left the classroom. In a fourth grade music class, several black boys "bebopped" to the admiring looks of their peers. One black boy walked with exaggerated hip shifts, the upper and lower torso moving in opposition; another boy walked about white shimmying his shoulder blades. A third sat snapping his fingers and then got up and performed a step-kick walking dance sequence. A fourth boy shook his arms and rippled his torso. As a sixth-grade class was going through the halls to the cafeteria, several black boys and girls performed a variety of dance movement phrases.

What specifically triggered the children's dance movements in the classrooms and halls was uncertain. For some children who find structured classroom activities incompatible with their capabilities or moods, dancing may be cathartic, a release of pent-up energy after adhering to a formal academic regime. In black folklore, the arts have a long history of providing solace and support. About black people black dancer Bessie Jones said, "We'd dance awhile to rest ourselves" (1972, p. 124).

Illustration 3. During recess outdoors on a warm sunny day, groups of black girls spontaneously organized dance cheers, ring-plays and line-plays that combine dance and song. Using the spatial form of children's dances probably of British origin and learned from white Americans, Afro-Americans meshed the African style of loose, flexible torso, extending and flexing knees with an easy breathing quality, shuffling steps, and pelvic swings and thrusts to create syncretistic dances of the sort that Bessie Jones and Bess Hawes describe as ring and line plays (1972, pp. 67–68). A leader either sang a phrase that the group answered or the leader led the performers. Movements accompanied and accented the song text or illustrated it. Hand clapping or other body percussion punctuated the performance to create a syncopated rhythm within the song and dance. In one instance, when a white girl wished to join the black girls in one of the dances, a black girl stepped back, put her hands on her hips, looked the white girl up and down about the hips and feet, and with a quizzical look and scowl said loudly for all to hear: "Show me you can dance!" Everyone watched as the white girl withdrew to the sidelines.

Later, a different white girl joined the "Check Me" ring play in which the name of each participant in the circle was singled out in turn, going to the right. One girl's name was called by the girl standing to her immediate left; she identified herself, sang a refrain, and then called on the next girl to her right.

> Check [clap], check [clap], check [clap]
> My name is Tina,
> I am a Pisces.

> I want you to [clap]
> check, check, check,
> to check out Bridgette.
> Check [clap], check [clap], check.
> My name is Bridgette. . .

When it was the white girl's turn to be called, the black girl just passed her by and called the next black girl. Rejected, the white girl called out, "I can do it, too!" No one paid attention.

In these dances, black pride, identity, boundaries, and neighborhood loyalty seemed to coalesce. By recognizing only blacks, the participants manifested in-group bonding in an arena in which they can excel, a response to the stressors of past white oppression and exclusion of black people. Their dancing suggests a way of coping with the stress: a future of racial separation possibly carried on as in the past—or even a reversal of power relations, blacks superior to whites. The white audience is put on its mettle. Perhaps the black girls' dances are similar to the slave animal trickster tales in which the weaker animal bests the stronger through its wits. The tales afforded their creators psychic relief, an arena of mastery, and a vision of a possible future.

Children often do not feel comfortable participating in arenas where they sense that they are not welcome, they are unlikely to perform well, or the competition is unfairly matched. Thus they stake out their own turf as ethnic minorities have always done. One consequence of the black dances is that the white children have the "outsider" status in informal children-delineated performance arenas at Pacesetter that blacks have had in broader arenas of life. By focusing on power through high energy dances, the girls suggest role reversal in the wider society. What the national context offers in prestige for whites, the local arena offers in recognition and power for blacks.

Commentary

From Africa to America, we have seen how dance is an autogenic medium to resist the negative effects of stress and to cope with stress in a remediative way. The dance may communicate messages of displeasure with situations that call for resolution. People of all ages express themselves through the dance.

It is fascinating that the Afro-Americans in Dallas had no direct contact with the Ubakala performers in Nigeria. Yet the pattern of protest through dance that is widespread and historically rooted in Africa appears to have survived in the new land.

Chapter 7
Revitalizing the Past to Recreate a Less Stressful Present: Asserting Ethnic Identity and Confronting Strangers

Groups may turn to their cultural roots when confronted with the stress of change and negative contact with other groups. These turnings to earlier practices usually mean a modification of them in light of the contemporary situation. Of course, change is always ongoing to some degree. Religious or secular responses that include dance may be attempts to revitalize what was perceived to have had positive benefit. Sometimes new dance forms evolve in which people reduce the stress of a sense of inferiority by identifying with the aggressor, accommodating rather than submitting, or resisting through defiant nonverbal expression. These dances provide arenas of self-affirmation and self-mastery in situations in which people feel they have lost political and economic power. The dancing is usually "framed," highlighted, or prepared for by religious offerings or other acts, such as using drugs, altering eating and resting patterns, and submitting to social isolation, that distinguish the everyday from the dance performance.

Bwiti

An example of a religious sect that developed in response to stresses and includes dance as a religious practice to meet life's travails is found among the Fang of Gabon. Bwiti, a 20th-century syncretistic cult or revitalization movement, draws upon both indigenous African and foreign Christian patterns and beliefs. The following information is drawn from Fernandez's extensive Bwiti study (1982). The dancing in Bwiti religious action and mythology stems from the Fang rather than the colonialist Christian tradition. Differing in some respects from the dances performed in other realms of Fang social life, skillful Bwiti dance performance is believed to obtain the blessing and benevolence of the dead. Leaders paint the feet of the members with a special paste to ensure flawless dancing.

Bwiti evolved in response to the Fangs' felt need for protection and revitalization as a result of the pressures of colonial domination and missionary evangelization along with the ennui prevalent among a previously turbulent people. The Fang experienced restricted personal expression and feeling states, and in the 1930s, Bwiti took a clandestine form because of objection to some of its practices.

Catalysts for Bwiti were harrowing threats of periodic famine, disease, and population decline coupled with occasional confrontations with missionaries or administrators. In one Fang "congregation," 30 out of 56 males had no children. Only Ekang's fourth and last wife produced two surviving daughters. In such infertile households, every conception is watched and a witchcraft accusation of one wife against the other in the event of miscarriage or the infant's early death is likely.

European contact led to increased scale of relationships in which "the reality of the far away has come to challenge what was previously the overriding reality of the near and the parochial. With Christianity came the challenge to the old traditional protectively benevolent powers of the below by the missionary message of divinity in the above" (p. 571).

The Bwiti cult is "a religious microcosm which 'placates' and 'reconciles' those who are troubled and separated in their relationships to one another, both gods and men. It satisfies by providing a whole experience for those to whom life does not provide enough of anything they feel they need, who feel they are not taking part or who, at best, feel they are allotted an insignificant part of the whole" (p. 4).

The "'knowledgeable ones' of Bwiti bring into being and reveal to their membership a 'pleasure dome' where they can be reconciled with the world and themselves and feel at home. It is a process of 'tying together' ... that which witches and sorcerers and the agents of the colonial world and simply modern times have rent asunder into that anxious isolated condition where men and women bereft of the solidarity of the group, the strength of the whole, are ... preyed upon" (p. 562).

This telling reason for joining Bwiti may well account for why dance "works" or is efficacious for many people: "I was a Christian but I found no truth in it. Christianity is the religion of the whites. It is the whites who have brought us the Cross and the Book. All the things in their religion one hears by the ears. But we Fang do not learn that way. We learn by the eyes" (p. 481). Fernandez points out, "Where there was a sense of bodily isolation and decay and vulnerability to circumambient evil, a burdensome sense of accumulating impurities, there is vigorous purifying engagement in ritual enactments followed by ecstatic transcendence of the corporeal" (p. 566).

The Fang represented the healthiness of flow in the social body by extension of their understanding of the importance of flow in the personal body. One act in Bwiti moves away from the quality of bad body to the quality of "clean body" or cleanheartedness. Because sexual appetite and indulgence are primary sources of "bad body", abstention and purity are sought in the ritual.

"It is regularly put forth by cult leaders that one of the purposes of the all-night dancing is to sacrifice to God and to the ancestors the sexual pleasure of the body (although at the metaphoric and symbolic level of culture activity there is plenty of sexuality being represented)" (p. 305). The all-night ceremonies end at dawn with dances that encircle the ancestors' welcoming hut and dances of compressed circles of "oneheartedness" performed in front of the hut, on the edge of the forest, and down in the center of the nearby stream. In a state of deep fatigue from the night's exertion, most of the members are pleased with their state of purity having rid their bodies of impurities through the vertiginous activity and copious perspiration (p. 532).

Sexuality has its place in Bwiti since a key purpose is the ritual inducement of fertility. The corporeal symbolism, carried out in the assimilation of the chapel itself to a body, appears in the men's entrance dances. "The men, following the women, arrive at the birth entrance of the chapel and halt there. The leaders place their hands on the thatch or the lintel piece above them. Then the entire group in close-packed formation backs up and comes forward again. At each successive surge forward they penetrate more deeply into the chapel. This continues until the male group is entirely within and ready to begin the circle dances. The ritual actions at the birth entrance are explained in various ways, but predominantly they are evoked as (1) the difficult birth of men out of this life into the spiritual world of the ancestors, and (2) the entrance of the male organ into the female body" (p. 389).

The Bwiti dance leader has assumed the name of the old Fang diviner and witch doctor whose task was to penetrate the unseen in favor of the afflicted. "The Bwiti *nganga*, by leading the membership fruitfully down the path of birth and death, does, in effect, like the *nganga* of old, enable them to penetrate into the unseen, to pass over into the land of the dead and, in so doing, to assuage their afflictions. Dancing successfully down the path of birth and death demands orderliness within the chapel. It demands the exclusion of agents of disorderliness such as witches and other errant supernaturals from the chapel" (p. 417).

Women participate in Bwiti. "And occasionally ritual dances other than the 'oneheartedness' dance go beyond complementarity to suggest interpenetration of the two parts into the whole" (p. 425).

The pounding chants, songs, and dances create an intense quality in performance. With variant meanings at different times of the evening, the *obango* dance generally refers to the turmoil of the soil as it either enters the body, at birth, or departs it, at death. "*Obango* has the meaning, if not of sexual passion, at least of ecstatic activity with fertile consequences." The women team dancers shake their buttocks, laden with sleigh bells which represent the child in the womb, "while their shaking of their buttocks is directly enticing" (p. 450).

Staying up the whole night is tiring; vigorous dancing, too, further exhausts Bwiti members. They take *eboga*, a crop common to the equatorial underforest that has psychotropic properties. In small quantities it helps to maintain wakefulness, sight, and physical energy. The *eboga* produces a euphoric insomnia. "Members often say that the *eboga* taken in this way also lightens their bodies so that they can float through their ritual dances" (p. 475).

Thus the ancestral Bwiti cult is a response to stress. In its ritual practices, especially the prominently featured dancing, Bwiti symbolically enacts wished-for resolution of personal and social difficulties. There is also the reality of people coming together and physically expelling accumulated tensions through the many hours of all-night dancing under a state of altered sensibility that results from the excitement, fatigue, and drugs.

American Ghost Dance

Native Americans have experienced years of stress from white political and economic domination. Defeat, the recognized inability to counteract the invaders and the ensuing poverty, seemed to fortify the Indians' faith to practice ritual designed to hasten world renewal. The Indians looked to the supernatural to accomplish what they could not do by themselves. Dance was part of a repeated florescence of Indian religious revivals that reaffirmed traditional values and enlisted ancient religious beliefs in periodic renewal of the world as a means of attempting to effect change. The Northern Paiute and peoples of the Northwest Plateau believed that ceremonies involving group dancing, a visible index of ethnic and political alliances and actions, had power to end the deprivation that resulted from defeat at the hands of whites and bring about a return to the earlier days of Indian prosperity, specifically the restoration of lost lands. In order to attract acculturated Indians, the Ghost Dance religion of the late 19th century incorporated Christian teachings of the millennium and the second coming of Christ. Modern transportation and communication spread the ideas (Stewart, 1980).

Moreover, there is an argument for the dance being a demographic revitalization movement (Thornton, 1981). The dance occurred at the time of a low in the American Indian population. Through disease, relocation, starvation, genocide, and social and cultural destruction, the American Indian population was decimated to an 1890 nadir of a mere 228,000 from an 1800 total of about 600,000. Virtually all smaller tribes participated in the dance, which was believed to return the deceased Indian people to life. A primary objective of the 1890 Ghost Dance (Mooney, 1896, p. 77) was the resurrection of the Indians' ancestors by returning the spirits of the dead from the spirit world.

Coast Salish Spirit Dancing

Aboriginal-style winter Spirit Dancing resurged in the 1970s among the Nooksack of Western Washington and more generally among other surrounding Coast Salish groups. Spirit Dancing had been declining since the advent of Christianity. The initial Indian-white contact had positive, rewarding exchange relationships. Christianity made inroads and intermarriage occurred. But full agricultural exploitation was incompatible with Indian hunting, fishing, and gathering. The onslaught of white-carried diseases hurt the Indians, who had little resistance. Then white attitudes turned against the Indians, whom they viewed as obstacles to progress. As a result, the Indians' aggressive adaptation evolved into passive nonparticipation in the white economy and poverty. The increased participation in the traditional ceremonial gives people an opportunity to affirm their worth as individuals and as Indians in a situation in which they have progressively lost economic autonomy and have had to depend on the white welfare system (Amoss, 1978).

The revival of Spirit Dancing is part of the trend toward celebrating ethnic traditions and joining cult-like religious movements. Spirit Dancing persists among the Indians because it expresses and reconciles major cultural values and is pleasurable. Like Pentecostalism and Shakerism, Spirit Dancing appeals to Coast Salish people, for it offers the opportunity for spontaneity and emotional release through a trance experience.

Prior to their contact with whites, the Indians exchanged food surpluses for wealth items through potlatch ceremonies. The Nooksack world view held that humanity was set apart from nature. In order to exploit the natural environment of salmon, saltwater fish, land animals, and edible roots and berries, a person needed to communicate with the supernatural realm. The vehicle for supernatural contact was a vision encountered with a somewhat personalized manifestation of the power that pervaded the wild realm of nature. This communication was ritually dangerous, and contact could be achieved only if the supplicant purged the taint of human existence by bathing, fasting, taking emetics, and submitting to social isolation.

Another aspect of the vision was a public symbolic presentation, usually in the form of a song or dance. The dance showed the strength of a person's power and thus marked the individual's role and status.

In contemporary religious belief the key spiritual entity is the "soul," an everpresent danger to its owner and others. Because the soul is light and easily dislodgeable from its owner, loss of the soul can cause illness to the owner as well as a person who has inadvertently attracted it (Amoss, 1978, p. 45). Consequently, children are not allowed on the floor of a dance house during a winter dance or permitted to get close to a new dancer.

Old patterns have changed. Instead of questing for power in adolescence and waiting five or ten years before dancing publicly, post-adolescent teenagers and older people now can become dance initiates. Instead of receiving an individualistic vision today, most participants now receive a vision that previously had been in the family. A tutelary of a deceased relative selects an appropriate candidate and troubles the individual until the person accepts and becomes a dancer. A spontaneous vision may come through sickness, sorrow, dreaming, or through dancers who grab individuals and infuse them with power.

Initiation creates a new social role for the candidate and mediates the contradiction between the principles of rugged individualism and of mutual support, cooperation, and interdependence of kin. Initiation begins with a rite of separation that lasts from four to ten days, during which the new dancer is purified and helped with his or her song. The following transition or liminal period lasts the rest of the dance season. Dancing is mandatory to avoid supernatural and social penalties. Often the words of the song and movements of the dance are stylized mimicry of the tutelary. The Indians believe illnesses respond to spirit dancing; magic spells may be used by dancers as protection in initiation and from hostile shamans.

Participants in the contemporary winter ceremonials belong to some local group, which in turn belongs to the larger dancing community. Seating in the dance house is organized according to village or reservation unit, as is the order of performance. The dance thus perpetuates intervillage ties, intensifies the bonds of the local unit, and promotes social solidarity and identity. A person needs his spouse's help to dance the spirit power properly. Thus the dance reinforces marital ties and the idea of family closeness as buffers to stressors.

The Nooksack require correct decorum in the dance. A dancer who falls, a drummer who errs and confuses a dancer, or a dancer who loses part of the dance costume, suggest ritual injury. Then the performer and his or her kin and their local group all lose face.

There are three kinds of invasion by an alien spiritual entity: a hostile spirit, friendly spirit, or strange soul who causes illnesses. Many dancers begin possession by crying or sighing in distress; the onset may cause a chest pain which dissipates when they dance. Entranced dancers perform a specific song and dance. The Coast Salish view the Spirit Dancer's trance as a special case of the pan-human capacity to seek altered states of consciousness.

Salish dancing allows catharsis, release of pent-up emotional tensions in a culturally valued and socially approved way that gives the performer a sense of mastery and autonomy. The self-confidence generated by the knowledge of being able to tap genuine supernatural resources offers the individual valid evidence of being special as an Indian in a world exclusive to the Indians.

The Gourd Dance

This dance, formerly performed exclusively by the Comanche, Wind River Shosone, Cheyenne, Arapaho, Omaha, and other warrior societies, has become popular with these groups and also with groups whose ancestors never performed it. The Kiowa and Comanche Group Dance Societies' invitational performances in the 1960s at the Tulsa powwow and other large intertribal urban powwows led to a momentum for the spread of the dance through the state of Oklahoma among 20 additional Indian groups and even beyond the state to Arizona and New Mexico. Howard (1976) suggests the dance provides a vehicle by which Native Americans can express their Indianness.

A Kiowa informant said about the dance, "It's just like prayer songs, it just makes you happy, and makes people feel good. . . .we want to help the people who may be in mourning and want to come back, or may be sick, or have troubles" (quoted in Howard, p. 247).

Singers sit in the center of the dance arena; male dancers sit on benches around the periphery. One bench is reserved for the female head dancer and her assistants. The other women dancers and spectators sit in folding chairs behind the benches. An invocation precedes the dance, which begins gradually with songs accompanied by dancers shaking their gourds softly in time with the music. The head male dancer and some of his friends rise and dance in place, shaking their gourds softly and treading quietly. They flex the knees on the loud beat and straighten them, sometimes with a slight bumping of the heels, on the soft beat. At times the dancers bend slightly forward from the waist making a swooping arm motion toward the floor. Other dancers gradually rise and join the performers as the beat picks up considerably. At the end of a song, signalled by a flurry of fast drum beats, the entire group of dancers raise their gourds high into the air and vibrate them. The tempo and excitement build up an electric atmosphere.

Danza de la Conquista

Originating in the states of Mexico's Queretaro and Guanajuato in response to the Spanish conquest in the 16th century, dance groups known as "concheros," "danza Chicimeca," "danza Azteca," and "danza de la conquista" persist. The groups, also called "crisis cults," are syncretistic attempts to create pride in their cultural identity and new forms of social integration in a changing milieu. Part of handling the stress of conquest and its lingering aftermath is identification with the aggressor (see Mitchell, 1956, on the Kalela dance in Africa for a similar pattern). Mostly from the laborer and shoeshine occupations, the dancers are at the low end of the socioeconomic scale. They adopt the nomenclature of the Spanish military hierarchy and perform dances reenacting the conquest. The dances were derived from the Spanish representations of Moors and Christians. Women, the aged, and children, as well as men, perform the warlike dances (Moedano, 1972).

Beni Ngoma

Popular in East Africa (urban and rural Kenya, Tanzania, Zambia, and Rhodesia, now called Zimbabwe), this dance is similar in some respects to the *danza de la conquista*. *Beni*, a popular, versatile team dance (*ngoma*) with essentially urban origins, has recognizable features of modernity (European dress, military band, drill, organization, and a hierarchy of officers with European titles), besides traditional competitiveness (1890–1970, Ranger, 1975). The dance is enmeshed in the stresses related to nearly 100 years of history (including colonial occupation, display of European military power, the devastation of World War I, the great depression and protest, the development of strike action, and the impact of World War II).

Beni, with elements of resistance, compulsion, and protest, is a medium of balancing emasculation and creativity, accommodation and independence. It is "one of a series of brass-band responses by people in a transitional period from pre-industrial to industrial society," comparable to the brass-band competitions of the Lancashire industrial village, band processions of 18th-century Jamaica or bands of Brazil (p. 6).

An indigenous form which selectively borrows from the powerful, *Beni* is an accommodation rather than a submission. This dance allows a display of self-respect and self-confidence in communal values based on locality, ethnicity, moiety, or class against others in a continuing tradition of communal dance competitions. These groups have elaborate ranks, displays of military skills, opportunities for innovation, achievement of high rank, and the exercise of patronage for high status.

Commentary

We have sketched some dances of peoples who felt stressed by the impact of domination by a more powerful group through colonialization or defeat in war. They suffered a loss of economic and social power. These stressors were besides those of life in general, natural disasters, and conflicting values about sexuality and individuality. Bwiti and *Beni* Ngoma dances from Africa and the Ghost Dance, Coast Salish Spirit Dancing, the Gourd Dance, and Danza de la Conquista from the Americas are examples of means to resist, reduce, or escape stress. Cathartic and avenues of altered states of consciousness, the dances may confront the stressors through physical and cognitive structuring in which the outcomes are favorable. Individuals find support in group dancing, which provides social cohesion, a kind of group therapy.

PART III

Illustrative Western Dance-Stress Relations

Having examined some of the palette of human experience in dance-stress relationships, we now turn to dance practices in contemporary Western society, particularly the United States. We will see how dance may be a means for people to resist, reduce, escape, or induce stress in the images and related activities that appear in social, educational, work, and therapeutic settings, theaters, and television. Now, through the widespread diffusion of television, dance can reach nearly the entire nation, whereas before, theatrical dance was the province of a narrow population of ticket-paying theater-goers.

Chapter 8
Playing with Stressors Onstage in Western Theatrical Dance

Modern Western society has advanced technology and a generally high quality of life that contrast with the situations of past societies, some Western minorities, and many non-Western countries. Yet, as members of the same species, people in modern society are affected by similar stressors related to life cycle vicissitudes and social exchanges. A prevalent leitmotif in the human record is that through dance themes such as death, sexuality, gender roles, violation of societal norms, and discrimination and oppression, dancers and observers attempt to cope with anxieties and fears. Kinetic discourse allows people to examine past, present, or anticipated events. The staged performance is pretend and therefore distant and less threatening than the real world.

When dance images are scrutinized to enlarge or illuminate the human outlook, the revelations about self or society may be like those in psychotherapy. The insight may move the individual to evaluate problems, consider resolutions, and act in a constructive way outside the dance setting. Indeed, it is this potency that leads many totalitarian countries to attempt to control dance and other arts, because they fear they will arouse the passions. Uninhibited ecstasy or its symbolic representations through contrast can remind the constrained how restricted they are. A political critique against a stress-inducing regime can be produced in dance texts not so much by an inherent or explicit political opposition as by a subversion of the artistic form.

Of course, much of dance is entertainment or play with form in and of itself, and thus for many dance participants is devoid of serious meaning and a diversion and escape from stress.

Contemporary stressors include death, discrimination and violence against minorities and women, limited opportunity, family perversity, detached love, gender conflict, and the dance career itself. This chapter will describe some illustrative dances that convey these themes and allow individuals to resist or reduce stress. Some of dances depict overlapping themes.

Death

After the tragic death of her two children, pioneer modern dancer Isadora Duncan choreographed "Mother," a poignant dirge for every mother who has lost a child. Martha Graham's "Death and Entrances" was inspired by the lives of the three Bronte Sisters and was also about Graham and her two sisters. Jerome Robbins dedicated "Quiet City" to Joseph Duell, New York City Ballet's principal dancer who committed suicide. The ballet ends with groups of dancers kneeling or standing in shadows.

Robbins's "In Memory of. . ." reveals young loving couples dancing together and then experiencing unrest. A young man who proves to be Death appears to claim one of the women, who struggles until he subdues her. George Balanchine's "Adagio Lamentoso" begins with three grieving women who dance barefoot and with loose hair. The mourners are joined by an ensemble to share with them reflections on the transitoriness of life and inevitability of death. "Dark Elegies," choreographed by Antony Tudor, suggests a communal ritual: through mourning, people cope with loss and death as a fact of life.

Eliot Feld's ballet "A Soldier's Tale" is about the horrors of war—including the pimp and prostitute who prey upon its men,, living and dead. Moving people to redressive action was the goal of Kurt Joss's 1932 anti-war ballet, "Green Table," still performed more than a half century later. It is an overt message about diplomatic duplicity, its path to war, and death. José Limon's "Missa Brevis" presents a chorus of dancers mourning in a bombed-out church.

Gerald Arpino's "The Clowns," choreographed in 1968 for The Joffrey Ballet and revived in 1987, is a parable about human survival in the face of nuclear war and its aftermath. The ballet explores cycles of rebirth and destruction adding a comic twist to the nightmarish theme: circus figures comment upon the ultimate ludicrousness of nuclear Armageddon. Technologically innovative in using huge clear plastic balloons and pillows, Arpino shows technology gone awry as it envelopes the clowns.

"Triumph of Death," Flemming Flindt's choreography of nude dancers performing to a rock score, dramatizes the manner in which human existence is threatened by environmental pollution, political tyranny and corruption, and cities contaminated by nuclear fallout.

Alvin Ailey's "Flowers" is about the doomed black-influenced white blues-rock cult singer Janis Joplin who became a drug addict. "Undertow," by Tudor, tells a story of a boy driven to murder. Crammed with nervous movement or urban restlessness and tension, the ballet presents scenes of brutal sex, hypocrisy, and other evils.

The plight of the American Indian, the slaughter and degrading violence against Indian women, is the theme of Michael Smuin's "A Song of a Dead Warrior." It has a cast of 31 dancers and spectacular effects—ghostlike sheriffs standing 20 feet tall and huge photographic blow-ups of bison. Smuin was inspired by the two-year occupation of Alcatraz by a group of Indian dissidents and the group leader, an Indian youth named Richard Oakes. He is portrayed as a young brave who dreams of ancestral rites and glory. Attending a reservation dance, he and his sweetheart are attacked by state troopers who rape and murder the girl. Overwhelmed, he becomes an alcoholic. We see the young man savagely beaten by pool hall thugs. Another ancestral vision comes to him. Inspired by his chiefly forebears, he rouses himself to fight, kill, and scalp the sheriff. His efforts are, however, to no avail; the troopers shoot him down.

(See comment on choreography about victims of AIDS in the section on homosexuality.)

Repressed Sexuality and Unrequited Love

As sexual beings who seek intimate relationships, people may be stressed by less than ideal outcomes. Tudor's "Pillar of Fire" is a tale of repressed sexuality. Hagar is on the verge of spinsterhood. She loves a man who is attracted to her younger sister. The tale of pathos eventually turns to Hagar's fulfillment. Robert Joffrey's "Remembrances" conveys the reverie of a composer's lost love through the mood of movement and music.

In Tudor's "Jardin aux Lilas," he reveals the pain of charming, gracious, affluent people bound by social conventions that restrict them. The dilemma is the misalliance of external material prosperity and social appearances and interpersonal feelings and misery. Caroline must forsake her true love, who is not of her social class, and enter into a marriage of convenience. Playing out secrets of stealthy approaches and sad partings, the ballet could be viewed metaphorically as a comment against any arbitrary constraints.

Americana, Sin, Perversity, and Alienation

With a merciless eye for Americana, Paul Taylor confronts duplicity and sexual perversity, from wife abuse and swapping to incest. Society's taboos surface as do the stresses of violating them. "American Genesis" is an evening-length biblical-historical-allegorical dance with period dance styles used to evoke period behavior. "The hillbilly Eden and the bouncy cakewalk and minstrel dancing in the final section, The Flood, convey to the audience something of the innocence of Adam and Eve in the Garden and the spirited irresponsibility of Noah's children. In Before Eden, Taylor sets up an air of seductiveness and sexual intrigue within the contained manners of a minuet. . . .

"Taylor takes some very unusual—you might say liberated—views of sex. . . . Women play male—parts—or the part of angels with male names. Adam and Eve try a *ménage à trois* with a fellow called Jake; then, after each one is left out in the cold while the others duet, they all decide to go their separate ways. Some early Americans are caught wife-swapping. As often as there's a character who goes naughty-naughty at some sexual innuendo, there's another character who's touting the benefits of Sin. Fun-loving Lilith's Child appears to inherit the hearth after the Flood, but stalking off close behind her is Lucifer, who first introduced Adam to her mother and, in the guise of Noah, later banned her from the Ark. . . .

"In West of Eden . . . he presents an orgy of lust, rape, and fratricide, with Cain and Abel being comforted impartially at the end by one Elder while the instigators—two other Elders who've previously been identified with Good and Evil—wash their hands of all responsibility. . . ." (Siegel, 1977, pp. 178–179).

Taylor's "Big Bertha," is "funny, macabre, garish, low-keyed, and provocative, all at the same time. It's about an all-American tourist family mesmerized into bestiality by a nickelodeon. . . .as the folks next door, Mr. and Mrs. B, come sauntering in with their cute daughter . . . a typical bloodless, 1946-nice family that doesn't have problems.

"Taylor puts a coin in Bertha's hand and as she begins to play, the family dance for each other, shyly at first and with polite nods of appreciation. Suddenly Big Bertha points her baton and Mr. B. goes goggle-eyed and slaps his wife. Then he's his old bland self; you hardly think it happened. But it did happen, and as Bertha pulls them into her power, the whole family turn into fiends. Mr. B. starts fondling his daughter, then drags her off to the bushes. She's shocked at first, but later she likes it. Mrs. B. meanwhile strips to her red undies and stands on a chair wiggling, something she has no doubt considered shameful all her life.

"As the orgy is building up, you remember that at the beginning of the dance you saw some exhausted red-clad figures crawling away, and you realize that Bertha is going to wring out the hapless B's the same way. She does" (Siegel, 1977, p. 213).

William Forsythe's ballet, "Say Bye-bye," without literally depicting physical abuse, is "aggressive, powerful and downright hysterical, both a pop ballet and a sharp commentary on the society. . . ." The entire atmosphere with loud sound, high-energy flinging movement and stylized lack of emotion among the characters "sports its alienation motif with the spiffiness of a new-wave rock group. Its powerful imagery is nonetheless a condemnation, not a glorification, of the mindless joyless gaiety it depicts." Onstage "six men, in white shirts and ties (but threatening in their tic of punching one black-leather-gloved hand into another) and six women in black, bounce, dance and neck as if there were no tomorrow. . . .a seventh woman, neurotic in her more conservative black dress . . . attempts to drown out the din. She screams 'Stop,' twitches and retreats to the symbol of [an] American car . . . parked in a corner of . . . [the] three-walled no-exit set. . . . The controlling image, actual and metaphoric, is of going nowhere. Abruptly, the ballet comes to an end" (Kisselgoff, 1982).

When the sexual revolution occurred in the 1960s, and expanded the range of partners with whom one could have intimate relations, sexual intercourse increased and became detached and impersonal. This created stress for some people. Robert Joffrey's intense, sexual, psychedelic ballet "Astarte" captures this ethos. From out of a seat in the audience, a male dancer reaches the stage, where he peels to his shorts and then engages in love-making with his partner—while on a huge billowing high screen above, a film gives an interpretive duplication of their actions onstage. The filmed images of the dancers are dematerialized, larger and more variable than life. In the duet, each partner seems to be responding to his or her own needs rather than the preferences of the other. Remote and unyielding she interacts with him in his desire. "For much of the dance they occupy separate areas of the stage, but even when they dance together, they have little sense of each other's space. Each one, separately, reaches a climax that is expressed in destructive fury. Each one, in a sense, rapes the other. When they move apart at the end, neither one has been satisfied or changed" (Siegel, 1977, pp. 122–123).

Anna Sokolow, a believer in the rebelliousness of modern dance, argues dances should draw upon stressful reality to provoke and shock. Her "Rooms" is about the loneliness and noncommunication of people in a big city. Chairs substitute for rooms, each dancer on one, isolated from all the others though physically close to them. "Opus 58" conveyed the feeling of the precariousness and violence of life. "Dreams" is about the nightmare of Nazi Germany.

"The Golden Years" is a bogus euphemism for the agonies of growing old in America. Although choreographers rarely concern themselves with this stressful problem, D. J. McDonald's "Nocturnes" depicts a middle-aged couple trying to recapture the romance of youth with bittersweet success. His "Grandfather Songs" includes different dancers taking turns portraying an elderly man whose life consists of listening to the radio in reverie.

Black Oppression

Because of segregation, blacks had their own theater circuits. When desegregation occurred, blacks began to present their choreography on stages along with whites. For example, Talley Beatty's "The Road of the Phoebe Snow" is evocative of the stressful life, youth, and death in the ghettos. So, too, is "The Black Belt." Donald McKayle's "Rainbow 'Round My Shoulder" is an angry dance of protest against the Southern black chain gang system. The men dream of freedom and women waiting on the outside.

"Morning without Sunrise" is Eleo Pomare's danced narrative about the people of South Africa. Imprisoned anti-apartheid leader Nelson Mandela's statement that "if things are not coming together, they are coming apart" inspired the choreography's scenes portraying the natural setting, unrest, revolution in the black township of Soweto, dying revolutionaries, and the poignant contribution of women fighters (Dunning, 1986).

Women's Liberation

Establishing one's sexual and gender identities are often stress-ful, especially when society is in a state of flux and traditional pat-terns are assaulted (Hanna, 1987b, 1987c, 1988c). In theater arts dance women had been portrayed as either virgin or whore; images in ballet conveyed male dominance through the traditional *pas de deux* in which the males support and manipulate women to allow them a greater range of movement. Female choreographers chal-lenge the typical male supremicist and female submissive scripts.

Through her dances, Isadora Duncan created an image of the female as a noble-spirited woman free to use her imagination and body as she wishes. Martha Graham, in the corpus of her choreography, dealt with dominance, unbridled female passion versus duty, attraction and repulsion, and submerged guilt and open eroticism. She made the women of such classic stories as Oedipus, Jocasta, and Oresteia human protagonists, where pre-viously they had been the pawns of gods and men. Graham por-trayed settler women of America's pioneer history in "Frontier" and "Appalachian Spring." In the dances of some female chore-ographers, heroic women take fate into their own hands, if only with an axe, like Lizzie Borden in Agnes de Mille's "Fall River Legend," who murdered her parents in order to free herself from their rules and strictures.

From woman's point of view, Graham's "Phaedra's Dream" dealt with the problems of a woman discovering that the man she loves is loved by another man, whose love he reciprocates. Her "Rite of Spring" portrays woman as sacrificial victim.

Senta Driver's choreography reversed dancers' traditional gen-der roles; we are used to seeing men lift women. Driver has her fe-male dancers lift and carry men and use their weight.

Women have traditionally been a sexual object that belonged to somebody. Dance has offered voyeuristic and erotic pleasure. Whereas feminists of Isadora Duncan's generation longed for sex-ual freedom and viewed puritanical repression as an obstacle to their emancipation, some feminists of the 1960s and 1970s feared the sexual revolution had not liberated women so much as made them more sexually available. Post-modern choreographer Yvonne Rainer's "Trio A" illustrates the removal of seductive involvement with an audience. The performers never confront the audience, and they avert their gaze.

Homosexuality

Being gay in American society has its stresses. In the United States homosexual sodomy was outlawed at the time of the Constitution and was a crime in every state until 1962. Twenty-four states and the District of Columbia impose criminal penalties. The AIDS (acquired immune deficiency syndrome) epidemic has engendered the current outbreak of homophobia. Note the Supreme Court decision *Bowers* v. *Hardwick* 478 U.S. (1986), which holds that there is no constitutionally protected right for homosexuals or heterosexuals to engage in sodomy. The gay liberation movement has had a startling turn in fortune. Homosexuality, after a steady climb from criminality to illness, to tolerated deviance, and to a life style celebrated in popular film and theater as well as theater arts dance, is reverting to public menace, symbol of death, and corruption of the soul.

Lesbians were not subject to the stress of being homosexual so much as being women. There were not court cases against them as against gay men (Bullough, 1976). Thus their danced exploration of lesbian themes is less prevalent than gays working through homosexual issues on stage.

On the fringe of society and receptive to the unconventional, the art world offers homosexuals an opportunity to express an aesthetic sensibility that is emotional and erotic, an insulation from a rejecting society, an avenue of courtship, and an arena in which to deal with homosexual concerns.

Choreographic motifs about homosexuality run the gamut: unhappy to joyous, masked to unmasked, lust to love, and male as woman. "Monument for a Dead Boy," choreographed by Rudi van Dantzig in 1965, was one of the first ballets to treat the making, life, and death of a homosexual. Parents, friends, sexual encounters, and psychic trauma are displayed in fragmentary narrative. "The boy, it seems, has been traumatized by a brutal display of parental coitus. He can't make it with a snaky seductress in blue; he feels dirty just thinking about it. He wants to go back to the days when he kissed a little girl among the hollyhocks, but this innocence is irretrievable and he turns to a young man for comfort. For this, the boy is taunted and gang-raped by a pack of school chums. With insult heaped upon injury, the boy kills himself" (Jackson, 1978, p. 38).

During the 1970s there were a number of ballets with *pas de deux* (or *trois*) for men as part of a larger work that showed the acceptance and beauty of homosexuality. For example, in "The Goldberg Variations" by Jerome Robbins, two boys dance together as two girls watch. Robbins hints at differing ways of love. "Weewis" by Margo Sappington for The Joffrey Ballet had a homoerotic male *pas de deux* that was about her husband's relationship with his best friend.

Some ballets are essentially homoerotic but pretend to be something else. Implicitly homosexual, "The Relativity of Icarus" by Gerald Arpino created a hullabaloo. Arpino denied the homosexual inference. Two male leads represent the mythic airborne figures of Daedalus and Icarus. Nearly naked they touch each other erotically in a cantilevered duet. Although they are supposed to be father and son, audience members saw no discrepancy discernible in age—easily achieved by make-up, costume, and movement—to make this believable.

Lar Lubovitch said AIDS was the motivation for his "Concerto Six Twenty-Two" (1985 French premier and 1986 United States), "because so many dancers have been stricken with AIDS, something the dance world doesn't own up to. . . . I felt that I wanted to show a version of male love on a platonic and high-minded level, to show the dignity of men who love each other as friends, that all men do have another man in their lives that they love so dearly, not in a homosexual relationship, but just all men, homosexual or heterosexual, have men that they love in their lives" (quoted in Parks, 1986, p. 56).

Transvestite dancing, long a component of the gay demimonde, surfaced from the semi-secret underground of clubs, largely frequented by homosexuals, to the stages of major theaters of the world capitals where drag ballet has played to standing-room-only crowds. Les Ballets Trockadero de Monte Carlo, one of several dance companies with the word Trockadero in their titles, has been a box office success throughout the United States. The drag act has been called misogynist. "All transsexuals rape women's bodies by reducing the real female form to an artifact, appropriating this body for themselves" (Raymond, 1979, p. 104). Yet most critics recognize the company as lovingly parodying the act of performance, specific ballets, and particular styles through informed in-jokes. Men show that they can do the same things that women can do in ballet and at the same time make a critical comment on what they should do.

Drag dance may be a means to cope with stress. Psychologists have pointed out that the pressure for a man to perform aggressively in a male role may be the cause for cross-dressing and related behavior (Brierley, 1979). In Western culture it is more acceptable for a woman to be like a man than the reverse. Travesty recognizes the feminine element in every man's nature and acknowledges that the difference between men and women is not so great. Travesty may thus reduce stress, create excitement, and relieve the pressure of sex role conformity. Sometimes a caricature of the image of the opposite sex is an attempt to demonstrate the right not to adopt an essentially heterosexual way of life; the parody calls attention to the cultural blueprint and the frequency with which it is disregarded. By being a lie, the duplicity of travesty is also a mockery of pre-existing sex roles.

Pain in Dance

About his "Footprints Dressed in Red" choreographed for Dance Theatre of Harlem, Garth Fagan said, "I wanted to say something about dancers as a community of workers and achievers, in the face of enormous pain. There's no pain in the world like the pain of dancers, going at it hour after hour, day after day, and then going home perhaps to a four or five-floor walk-up—it's excruciating. . . . The red . . . is meant to refer to the pain and blood that's a given in black culture all throughout the world" (quoted in Kriegsman, 1987, p. F10).

Commentary

Although some dance participants perceive theatrical performance merely as entertainment and consequently a means temporarily to escape stress, dance has even greater potential. Through the performance of themes related to the trials and tribulations of life, dance may be a means to resist or reduce stress. Choreographers, dancers, and observers may resist stress by anticipatory socialization as described in Chapter 5. Themes of death, sexuality, gender roles, violation of societal norms, and discrimination and oppression are held up to scrutiny. These issues may provide catharsis, albeit through spectator empathy, and thus reduce stress. Participants in the theatrical event of dance performance may gain distance and insight that move them to resolve some of their problems. Alternatively, the themes portrayed in dance may scrape raw nerves and induce stress.

Chapter 9
Stressors in Pursuing the Western Dance Career

Classical ballet dancers must study from the age of eight for 10 years before they might—just might—move in a way that is interesting and beautiful to watch. As professionals we work 12 hours a day for six days a week. We inhabit an environment of order, routine, discipline, beauty and youth. Our obsessive preoccupation with physical perfection is the external result of a deep, silent, and very private spiritual commitment.

Thus wrote Toni Bentley (1986), a member of New York City Ballet, one of the world's most prestigious dance organizations. Her remarks about a demanding career were in response to the suicide of a friend and colleague in the dance company, Joseph Duell, who took his life on February 16, 1986. The road to becoming a professional is filled with stressors. And among those who make it to the top, not all can cope with the demands of the field and their aspirations in or outside it (Hager, 1978).

Yet, ballet and other forms of dance create illusionary worlds and may provide an escape from the everyday world's stresses and an outlet for releasing tension. For renowned prima ballerina Gelsey Kirkland, who danced with New York City Ballet and then American Ballet Theatre, dance offered a convenient way to avoid her father, a writer who had fallen upon difficult times and had turned to alcoholism and family fights. Escaping from home to ballet also "gave me a creative arena in which to vent my rage. . . . If I was not able to control my social world, I could at least begin to co-ordinate the movements of my own body. By devoting myself to the discipline of dance, I was able to establish a measure of control that was otherwise lacking in my life, or so it seemed" (1986, pp. 26–27). She was bound to "those feelings and ideas that came with each breakthrough in my understanding" (p. 212). Mikhail Barysh-nikov, ballet and movie star, said, "The stage is a form of opium for me—a psychological feeling I must have, I cannot be without" (quoted in Kirkland, 1986, p. 212).

This chapter will discuss some of the stressors associated with becoming and being a professional dancer: attitudes toward the dancer, roadmaps for the career and career transitions, perform-ance anxiety, cooperation and competition, physical injuries, food and weight, improvisation movement and contemplative creativ-ity, and economic survival.

Society's Attitudes toward the Dancer

Twenty-six years prior to Duell's unexpected death, Agnes de Mille, renowned dancer and choreographer, drew candid observa-tions and conclusions from a lifetime spent in the classroom, re-hearsal hall, and theater to write a book called *To a Young Dancer: A Handbook for Dance Students, Parents, and Teachers*. Much of what she says still pertains and is relevant to stress-related matters.

Dancers have always moved in an aura curious and provocative if often at the same time despised. They are widely discriminated against, and although their appeal at the moment seems to be uni-versal, with the figure of ballet girl a constant in advertising, laws and social custom are slow to reflect this enthusiasm. Dancers still cannot get leases or insurance as readily as other people, and in England they are not permitted to rent cars. The theater itself dis-criminates against them, and distinctions are made in dressing rooms, courtesies and comforts, fees and billings. A dancer who wishes to better his terms materially must become known as an actor even at the cost of subordinating his true metier. This still pertains in an age when dancers break theatrical frontiers and set creative standards unmatched before (1960, p. 4).

In Europe dance was not considered a proper, respectable profession for ladies and gentlemen. However, working-class youth welcomed the training, livelihood, pension, and opportunity for glory. Contrary to the private enterprise nature of dance in the United States, governments in other countries often subsidize major, and sometimes minor dance companies, and schools, and they maintain dancers as civil servants, cared for with salaries and pensions and recognized the whole of their lives. The Soviet Union, China, the United Kingdom, France, Sweden, Denmark, and Cuba are among the countries whose governments support dance. (See Panov, 1978, on stresses unique to dancers in the Soviet Union.)

De Mille writes about dancers in America whose lives are not so securely ordered as they are in places with government support.

They are looked upon with all the doubts visited on any vagabond. Parents would certainly hesitate about permitting a daughter to marry a dancer, while the thought of a son embracing the profession causes such acute dismay as has on occasion resulted in outright disinheritance. There is still a general reluctance to ask dancers into nice homes except on the most transient basis and prompted by curiosity (1960, p. 4).

Lincoln Kirstein, co-founder with George Balanchine of the School of American Ballet and the company it feeds, the New York City Ballet, of which he is General Director, said, "When I grew up, a father would rather see his son dead than a dancer" (quoted in Temin, 1982). Choreographer Brian Macdonald said his family wanted him to be a lawyer, and his refusal was tantamount to prompt disinheritance: "The day I joined the National Ballet of Canada in 1951, my father changed his will. He died without ever changing it back" (quoted in Stoop, 1984, p. 62). Of a younger generation, Douglas Dunn, dancer/choreographer trained in art history at Princeton, said his parents, both doctors, were not happy with his career choice. A 1980 "pulse reading" on attitudes toward dance came from Ronald Reagan's campaign headquarters: the politicians concerned with reactions of the Moral Majority seemed embarrassed that as *The Washington Post* (June 25, 1980) put it, "While his dad does the White House waltz, Ronald P. Reagan, 22, is jete-ing for the Joffrey II Dancers."

Bentley put it this way: "We really are a funny class of society—we come from all backgrounds, from mailmen's kids to doctors' and lawyers' kids. We are uneducated, apolitical and generally amoral—except where dancing is concerned. Because dancing is now at such a peak of popularity, we are accepted by the world as desirable social beings, but we are really pretty alien. We are also performing, even on social occasions—playing the role of the dancer. We don't know what else to be" (1982, p. 20).

In the minds of the broad public, female dancing has been associated with moral laxity; male dancing has been similarly associated, especially with homosexuality. Despite the receptivity of the art world to deviance from what is generally accepted in the broader society, some dancers make efforts to keep their sexual lives private.

Individuals who go into the occupation of dance as part of an effort to enhance self-esteem (related to a faulty body image and a continuing re-enactment of approach-avoidance relationships with a parental figure) may experience stress if they come from or work in a milieu which has negative stigma associated with dancing. This paradoxically lowers self-esteem. The dancer partially fulfills a need for public approval through a process which simultaneously exacerbates that same need (Halpern, 1981). Choreographer/dancer Blondell Cummings spoke at the Dance Theater Workshop's critical seminar "Talking about Sex and Dance," November 2, 1986, about the conflict she experienced between her strict religious upbringing and the demands of her art. She had been asked to bare her chest.

Female dancers, as other working women, desire to achieve and, at the same time, fear disapproval for achieving. Some struggle to compete in the workplace with men while simultaneously fulfilling the role of wife/mother (Braiker, 1986).

There are several approaches to upgrading the status of dancers and destigmatizing the profession. University dance programs, comparisons of dancers to athletes, the involvement of a range of occupational groups (including policemen and elected officials in dance (as former New York City Ballet principal Jacques d'Amboise does in staging annual performances, some of which are nationally televised), and superstars' six-digit incomes help to overcome the reservations people have about dancers. Performers like Rudolf Nureyev, Mikhail Baryshnikov, and Natalia Makarova are celebrities and respected.

Ballet student, teacher, and anthropologist Daniel O'Connor observed how dancers dealt with the problem of homosexuality. A male dancer (straight or gay) might handle the issue with nondancers by first acknowledging the stereotypical image and then establishing himself as an exception. He does this by revealing, for example, that he has a girlfriend, he finds gays disgusting, or his love of ballet makes him "put up" with gay men. Other men offer information that would lead an outsider to believe the stereotype of the male dancer is unfounded. Another strategy is dressing like a successful businessman or gentlemanly scholar and communicating machismo through body language.

Most people today go into professional dance out of a passion, not for the rewards of financial security and stability, the conventional rewards of an occupation. Motivation to dance professionally often includes the satisfaction of achieving what others want to do, try to do, but cannot do well. Dancers may perform for us and in place of us. Performance tends to catapult the successful dancer to heights of exhilaration. Yet, there is no guarantee of success, even after a huge expenditure of time, effort, and money in training, self-discipline, and sacrifice.

Choreographer and Dance Company
Manager Behavior toward Dancers

The choreographer/artistic director often has an absolute monopoly on taste and creative control and considers the dancer an expendable commodity. Ballet dancer Gary Chryst noted that a choreographer knows a person at 18 and then the person is not 18 any more. This, too, creates stress for the growing person who needs more challenge (Chryst, 1986, p. 44).

Kirkland comments on Balanchine, who "assembled steps that were supposed to have been predetermined by God and humbly described himself as an instrument of divine will. His word was holy" (1986, p. 50). Moreover, "he sought to replace personality with his abstract ideal of physical movement. . . . The interpretive stamp of a dancer threatened to mar the choreographic design of the master" (p. 45). The master was not to be questioned. His dictim was "Just dance" (p. 46). Although Balanchine was famous for describing ballet as "Woman," and the ballerina inspired him, an inspired approach to dancing for his dancers was almost unthinkable. "He often said, 'There is no such thing as inspiration.' Our devotion made us dependent on him for ideas and psychological motivation" (p. 48).

According to the aesthetic code of Balanchine and his collaborator composer Stravinsky, "the human condition was reflected primarily through animal and mechanical imagery, to be realized through the senses by way of instinct and imitation. . . . Stravinsky put it, 'An artist is simply a kind of pig snouting truffles'" (p. 68).

Enforced infantilism stresses thinking dancers. Kirkland wrote, "The problem I have experienced in the world of ballet is that free discussion has been inhibited by idol worship and prejudice, by the pressures for success, by the fears of failure within the profession of dance. . . . The difficulty with Balanchine, as with many of the Russian men I have known, was that he did not think women were capable of engaging him with ideas. . ." (p. 67). Yet, "I knew that my dance was both an act of will and a means of expression. Ballet was the only link that I had ever been able to make between thought and action. Simple logic told me that I had to make the same connection on stage. I had to find a way to break through the barrier that separated art and reality" (p. 118).

Kirkland had a zeal for perfection, yet she was filled with passivity and guilt instilled by the ballet culture. She feared to challenge the prevailing aesthetic and popular authority figures. Rage festered inside her (p. 175). When she felt like a failure, she tried to reassert control. "I began to starve myself . . . I was trying to disappear, to deny my physical existence altogether . . . I wanted to empty myself out completely. Purification and punishment seemed to go hand in hand" (p. 90). *Anorexia* is the morbid pursuit of weight loss which can lead to a state of starvation. *Bulima*, a cycle of eating binges followed by purges, is another destructive stress response, an attempt to gain control, "blot myself out" (p. 166). Ultimately, the stress of the milieu that demanded conformity, unquestioning slavery, led her to cocaine: "Only the drug enabled me to work and dance that way—without conscience" (p. 231). Cocaine enabled Kirkland to "avoid the misery, the agony that existed in a theater that rejected perfection in favor of expediency and box office receipts" (p. 244).

Ballet company mentality of prolonged immaturity and dependency makes dancers, without strong emotional support from family or authority figures, susceptible to bodily abuse. Gifted dancers who are pushed within the company are placed under unrelenting pressure. According to Kirkland, two out of ten dancers were trying to starve or poison themselves to death. The companies accept neither the responsibility nor the financial burden of providing professional counseling and care for those dancers.

Balanchine did not like his women dancers dating; he wanted their sole devotion. "Motivated more by jealousy than concern, Balanchine encouraged an atmosphere that was a mixture of convent and harem" (p. 40). To be sure, sometimes sexual energies were siphoned off in dance. However, the permissive attitudes of the times were at odds with the discipline of dance and its spartan work ethic. "Under the strictures imposed by Balanchine sex was about the only weapon his dancers possessed. Defying the sexual taboo makes it seem possible to escape his domination" (p. 41).

Managers disregard the dancers as humans subject to physical and mental trauma in spite of their high energy and resilience. Although he recognized children's physical vulnerability, "in actual practice, Balanchine and his teachers unwittingly encouraged young dancers to self-destruct, rationalized as part of the sacrifice that must be made to the art. The speed and shortcuts that he built into the training process called for physical cheating in which the dancer distorted the body to deliver the position or step that Balanchine demanded. The risk of injury was ignored. I watched many of my friends become casualties and fall by the wayside" (p. 34). "Misguided and caught between excessive demands for turnout and pointe, my feet had already begun to deform. At the age of eleven, I came down with a severe case of bunions. Many of the teachers had the same malady, caused form years of strain placed on the foot. It was said that Balanchine cherished the aberration of line induced by bunions, that they contributed to the impression of winged feet. . . .the discomfort soon became so crippling that I was forced to see a doctor. . . . He advised me to quit ballet. . . . I danced through the pain and compensated as well as I could. At age twelve, the tendons in my ankles became acutely inflamed. I tried to inure myself to the aches and twinges. This became the standard operating procedure for all injuries throughout my early career" (p. 35).

Balanchine's insensitivity toward the dancer's well being is put thus: "Dear, you're young. Young people don't have injuries. Go home and read fairy tales. Try little red wine. . . . You need nothing but this place. You don't need anybody else; you don't go anywhere else. You have a beautiful theater here. You come in the morning. When you don't work, you go into studio by yourself; you do releves. You must stay here all day; you go home, drink little red wine. That's all you need" (p. 51). On tour with New York City Ballet, Kirkland became emaciated, green, and seriously ill in Moscow. Balanchine insisted she perform. She had no replacement, it was opening night, and there were important people in the audience. Balanchine gave her a "vitamin" so that she would "feel much better" (p. 96).

Roadmaps

Knowledge about the trials and tribulations of a dance career certainly helps prepare an individual for its perils and alleviate some of the anxieties of the unknown. Even the stars are often surprised. Patrick Bissell of the American Ballet Theatre reflected:

> I thought it would be a hell of a lot more glamorous. I'm finding out you're always beat, you're always bushed. You don't have time to feel glamorous. I thought, just a few years ago, that dancing the roles I'm doing now would be a lot of fun and games, and New York would be endlessly exciting, and there would be a lot of terrific parties. Now I've found out that when there are parties, I don't go because I'm too tired (quoted in Jacob, 1981, p. 96).

He met the stresses of relentless pressures with sex and drugs (Kirkland, 1986) but died at age 30.

A more recent work than de Mille's is Ellen Jacob's *Dancing: A Guide for the Dancer You Can Be* (1981). Every year *Dancemagazine* publishes an annual that lists current information for training, performance, and related resources. In *Dancemagazine* articles and Jacob's book, one can read about possible choices of forms of dance and schools, criteria for evaluating one's choices and progress, matters of health, places to live and eat that are economically reasonable, issues of physical security in strange cities, steps toward launching a performing career, and success stories of career dancers.

The May 1986 issue of *Dancemagazine*, for example, has an article on "Health: Doctors for Dancers." It points out that throughout the United States, clinics and hospitals provide special services for the physical and psychiatric health of dancers. There are often special days and hours and reduced rates for dancers. New knowledge, therapies, facilities, and professions have emerged to provide additional ways and sources to treat dancers. Services for dancers are frequently a division of a center's sports medicine clinic.

New York City is the dance capital of the United States, perhaps the world. Consequently, aspiring dancers seek to study and perform there. The city has its special stresses. Sara Maule, who came from the West coast and joined American Ballet Theatre, remembers this reaction:

I found the hugeness of everything in New York overwhelming. I remember looking at all the buildings, with all their windows and thinking: *There's a person behind each one.* San Francisco was a cosmopolitan city, but New York was still a shock. In San Francisco I had teachers who took care of me and nurtured me. What was most traumatic about New York was the anonymity. There were so many dancers, all with different reasons for being there, all going their separate ways. There were so many people in class that the teacher was more impersonal too. Joining Ballet Theatre helped. Once you're in a union company the pay is good and you have good job security. But that in itself was a shock. Ballet Theatre was such a big company—there were so many people, and everyone fighting to make it. It was a family, but after my experience in San Francisco, a big, impersonal one (quoted in Jacob, 1981, p. 285).

Kirstein compares the excitement of ballet to the excitement of battle with its physical risks. "Dancers are always at hazard, always in an extreme situation. When your body is in danger, it illuminates a whole other capacity. It gives you new muscle. It throws you back on yourself" (quoted in Temin, 1982).

The life style of ballet is similar to that of a religious order and it fulfills similar psychological needs: both religious orders and ballet institutions have a similar mortification of flesh, adoration of saints, canonization of the highly esteemed, a representation of something larger than the individual, and insistence about giving up the self and world for a greater good. The company acts as an exterior superego driving the dancers, their individuality subdued (Mazo, 1974, pp. 105–106). The spate of autobiographies of dancers with major companies reveal dimensions of the ballet lifestyle that can sensitize the novice.

Careers and Career Transitions

As noted earlier, professional dancing is a short-term occupation. Dancers reach the end of their careers usually at mid-life, about 35 years of age when the body instrument shows decline. Moreover, as sociology professor David Earl Sutherland put it, "Dance is a career dedicated to systematic downward mobility, in opposition to the general American value upon upward social mobility" (quoted in Weston, 1982, p. 11).

"All dancers wage a losing battle against gravity and time, their bodies the instruments of betrayal in a world obsessed with youth and fairytale illusion. Airborne grace and quicksilver technique come of daunting offstage labor and a singular passion for physical perfection. With the years, the dancer's artistry gains nuance and depth, yet, paradoxically, speed, power and flexibility begin to wane" (Solway, 1986). It is stressful when older dancers get the tip-off: "They are not cast in ballets they always danced, or when they are asked to teach their roles to younger dancers. 'If you're not in a new ballet every other season, you're edited out,' says Francisco Moncion, whose longer career as a leading dancer with City Ballet began in 1946" (ibid.).

Karen Kain, a leading dancer with the National Ballet of Canada, said, "The very mention of retirement strikes terror in most dancers." At 35, she has "yet to grapple seriously with the topic personally, but confesses that its inevitability haunts her. President of the newly opened Dancer Transition Center in Toronto, created to help dancers adjust to retirement, she says, 'Like everyone else, I want to go on dancing forever, but I know the day is going to come when I will have to be doing something else. You're terrified that nothing will ever give you the fulfillment that dancing has given you" (ibid.).

Most professional ballet dancers forgo college. In 1960, de Mille knew of only six choreographers of different dance forms with degrees: Birgit Cullberg, Katherine Dunham, Sybil Shearer, William Bales, Myra Kinch, and herself. Without university degrees, career transitions are often traumatic if a dancer does not choose or have opportunities to teach in a studio, choreograph, or work in another capacity for a dance company or arts organization. Because modern dancers commonly have university education, it is easier for them to segue into university dance departments.

Credentials make a difference, although they are worthless in the absence of a solid track record. Yet, Carolyn Adams, former dancer with Paul Taylor, said sometimes the track record can be a liability in the sense of raising questions as to the ability to shift style (1986).

"Tunnel vision," the refusal of dancers to acknowledge the reality of a transitory career until it is over because they are devoted solely to the physical and aesthetic demands of dancing, ultimately creates stress. San Francisco Ballet dancer Victoria Morgan spoke of the strict discipline that directors demand from their dancers: "You get into this frame of mind where you just want to say 'Yes, sir' and do exactly what the director tells you to do because he has total control in this little world. Dancers in this situation end up not trained to think for themselves." Richard Le Blond, Jr., president of the company, took up the point: "Perhaps dancers live in a world where they're not permitted to reach emotional maturity, and that really comes out in the language itself. What other profession calls adult artists 'kids'? What other profession refers to people who have been practitioners of their art and in their thirties as 'boys' and 'girls'?" (quoted in Weston, 1982, p. 11).

Performance Anxiety, Cooperation, and Competition

The dancer's life is one of continual cooperation, performance, and competition. Training itself is a kind of performance. Students compete for the teacher's attention and approval (Forsyth and Kolenda, 1966). The dancer always depends on others' evaluations: teachers, judges at schools, auditions, and other competitions, choreographers who select dancers for special roles, and audiences, including those special members, the critics (Hanna, 1985). There is always pressure, even when evaluators build up a budding talent. Expectations cannot always be met.

Victoria Bromberg of the New York City Ballet reflected upon her experiences at the School of American Ballet:

The competition at SAB wasn't necessarily a bad thing, because it prepared you for the competition and discipline in the company. It's part of your training. You learn how to keep yourself together, as you must if you want to stay in the company. There is no probation period in the New York City Ballet as there is in the Paris Opera, where they give you a year to pull yourself together if you let yourself get out of shape or fall down on technique (quoted in Jacob, 1981, p. 297).

Although performance is the goal of professional dance, appearing in front of an audience can be scary (Aaron, 1986). Stage fright is a state anxiety, a deviation from the person's usual level or trait anxiety.

Performance means being on the spot. You are "out there." You are vulnerable. You are naked. Everything shows. There is no place to hide, because even if you seek it, then that is what shows. So there is no escape. This is at once the magic of performance and the terror of it. It is both what attracts us to it and which induces us to make such statements as, "I will never perform again." It is our banner and our hara-kiri sword. In our times, the sense of being on edge has been heightened by two factors. One is the separation that has been created between performance and audience. It can be a paralyzing split. The second is the ethic of individuality, which produces aggression and intensifies the frozen quality of the performance arena (Rockwell [Nadel], 1984).

Dancing in front of an audience involves risk—a slip, misstep, gesture offbeat, forgetting what is supposed to be done. Fear of failure is most troubling. Dreadful apprehension may also occur when the theme of the dance threatens to become real, that is, the roles the dancers enact are too close to the performer's immediate personal life experiences. For novices, stage appearances are frightening because they are inexperienced. Some professional dancers, however, have stage fright all their lives with anxiety attacks of jitters, sweating, shaking, feeling faint, needing to use the toilet. Fear of the audience activates the flight-or-fight mechanism.

Yet the stress of stage fright also has beneficial effects. It may lead to the performer's heighted awareness, sensitivity, and drive to succeed that lead to excellence.

Why do some dancers get nervous before a performance while others experience no discomfiture? The answer may lie in their training experiences. Youngsters who have a large proportion of successes develop confidence. Those who have many failures often develop expectations of further mistakes and consequently experience negative stress. For young performers, some teachers do not discuss stage fright because they believe that fear is contagious. Others talk about it in a supportive way to reassure performers that stage fright is not unusual. There are, said psychoanalyst Sanford Weisblatt, "good psychological reasons for teachers to wait until they have something to respond to from students. The essence of this has to do with the risk that the student will unconsciously experience the teacher as wanting the student to experience anxiety or suffering" (quoted in *Medical Problems*, 1986, p. 13). Some excitement evokes alertness and an attempt to do one's best.

The process of attending a conservatory requires an audition before a group of critical people who provide negative comments. The audition situation continues for jobs after one's schooling. That is, there is a series of events in the performance career, each with negative reinforcements. The negative aspect of competition may produce a bad self-image and tensions and anxieties. Charles O. Brantigan, a cardiovascular surgeon who trains surgeons and occasionally performs music, contrasts the training and life of a performer in the arts and a performer in surgery: "With our surgeons we try to create an expectation of success. Most of the musicians with whom I am associated have an expectation that there is going to be a problem. . . . The surgeon in training first has the opportunity to observe an operation. When he gets the idea of how everything goes, his professor turns part of it over to him. Over the years it's a sequence of gradually increasing responsibility. If the guy gets in trouble, he doesn't get booed by the audience or criticized by the jury. There's an expectation of success, with someone there to make sure it's successful" (*ibid.*, p. 14). Of course, the process of getting into medical school is a highly competitive one. And mistakes in surgery can eliminate surgery or even other forms of medicine as a career.

When she was at the School of American Ballet, Kirkland said, "The nature of my compulsion was such that I danced in my sleep. The entire household was sometimes awakened by loud thumping sounds coming from my room. The source of the disturbance was discovered to be the rhythmic blow of my foot against the wall next to my bed as I performed *grand battements*, a step that might be misconstrued as the classical version of a chorus line kick. Even in my sleep, I was struggling to perfect the technical execution of the step" (1986, p. 30).

She noted that "the vicious pressure of competition invariably turned dancer against dancer" (p. 37). The success of one dancer may be the failure of another. Moreover, the success is not something static. A dancer is continually being tested.

Bentley took her first ballet lesson at the age of three. In her journal she wrote about her School of American Ballet audition eight years later:

> Finally her name was called. She marched with her mother into the office. Yes, she was lovely; yes, they would take her; yes, she was thin, graceful and lovely. . . . She was thrilled, thrilled by a success that she had not planned. In fact, until the moment she realized that she had been singled out from the other children, she had never before known the feeling of success. It was a happy feeling. She also realized somewhere below the surface that her success was inevitably connected with the failure of others (1982, pp. 6–7).

However, five months after her admission, the school had doubts about her talent, future, and feet. It was not certain that she would be allowed to continue after the first year. "She was angry.

Very angry. She threw her beloved toe shoes down the incinerator. Her parents were shocked at the apparent pain she felt" (*ibid.*, p. 7).

She succeeded in the school and during her seven years moved to the top. Others had been weeded out. Some grew too tall, fell in love, or went to college. During her last year she injured her foot and could not dance for three months. Upon returning to class, Balanchine was there to select girls to perform the ballerina parts in the school's workshop performance, the pinnacle in the students' career. He chose her to learn Princess Aurora in "The Sleeping Beauty." After six months of rehearsal, she slipped the week before the performance. Despite sitting for the last week of rehearsals in a chair with a black and blue ankle packed in ice, on the morning of the performance she danced. "She felt no pain at all. She was injured for a month afterwards. But she had danced, and she had triumphed. She was not going to give up the chance of a lifetime" (p. 8).

Bentley realized her dream and joined the company. What is more, she was chosen for special parts. And then one day instead of her name being seen alone, it was seen with others. "So perhaps the road to Ballerina Land was not going to be as straight as I had planned. . . . It was devastating. The straight lines . . . zigzagged all over the place. Going forward used to mean going forward. I think now that it means going backward" (p. 12).

At the age of 22, dancing was not serving her purpose. "Unless you're out there on the big stage *alone,* you've no chance to communicate and know you're being successful" (p. 14). Experiencing a stagnating career, she reflected: "What can I feel but at some sort of ending? . . . I suppose I should be happy I am still young enough to begin again, but I've no money, no lover, no future I can see, only the same ballets, seasons after seasons. . . . What else is there? There is the example of the good survivors, those who bounce back over and over. They have an outside life and outside interests, so when dancing fails, they can keep themselves occupied in a nondestructive way and wait for the will to dance to emerge again of its own accord" (pp. 96–99). Bentley took a leave of absence from the New York City Ballet and then returned. She had to leave to see what she left—"the bliss of total immersion, total concentration in dancing. . . . I have a joy and an energy . . . I am a dancer" (pp. 148–149).

When dancers are supposed to master new dance material that is incompatible with previous ways of moving, they may experience anxiety and depression (Predock-Linnell, n.d.). A continual stressor for the choreographer and dancer is the popular belief that, as David White, a dance producer put it, "You are only as good as your last review" (quoted in *Update Dance/USA* 2 (5): 2, 1982). The choreographer and dancer are treated as commodities: when talent burns out, another fresher model is waiting to star. Kirkland's autobiography, *Dancing On My Grave* (1986), attests to how the stressors of dance in America lead to self-destructive acts. Dancers push themselves to the limit. The intensity of performances, even on top of physical injury, has at times been heightened by artificial resources of energy.

Choreographers, the creators of dances, may experience anxiety about being able to produce. Perfectionists worry about their work measuring up to their high standards. Pressures of deadlines and limited resources intensify the situation. Choreographers are risk-takers and fear failure. They must innovate within the dictates of American aesthetics. However, too much innovation is damaging to others in challenging the status quo and losing audiences unfamiliar with or unreceptive to the avant-garde. The positive features of creators as unique and marvelous have their negative counterparts: independence/loner-outsider, questioner/troublemaker, flexible/uncommitted.

Physical Injuries

Dancers may choose not to seek help with injuries out of fear that the doctor will tell them not to use an injured body part for a period of time. The conclusion of this book discusses some of the warning signals of injury and guidelines for their prevention.

Food and Weight

Thinness, the current reigning aesthetic for ballet and much of modern dance, contributes to health by placing less stress on vital organs during strenuous activity, to fleetness, and to being lifted easily. Eating what one likes is not always compatible with staying in shape. The competition between one's culinary desires and one's career demands create a range of stresses.

Ballet choreographers and directors—"almost always male—mold ballet's young women to the idea of feminine that equates beauty and grace with excessive thinness," an aesthetic that is punitive and misogynist (Gordon, 1983, p. 173). Balanchine set the standard. Kirkland reports (1986, p. 56): "He halted class and approached me for a kind of physical inspection. With his knuckles, he thumped on my sternum and down my rib cage, clucking his tongue and remarking, 'must see the bones'. . . . He did not merely say, 'eat less'. He said repeatedly, 'Eat nothing'."

Relentless pursuit of the unnatural "ideal" female body arrests puberty, imbalances hormones, contributes to hypothermia and low blood pressure, and invites bone injury. Moreover, this pursuit often leads to psychosomatic disorders of starvation, vomiting, and the use of laxatives (Vincent, 1979). Anorexia and bulima are interconnected with injury. These eating disorders are also misplaced efforts to control one's destiny.

Medical doctor Douglas Anderson notes:

Ballet students collectively comprise the highest risk group for the development of serious eating disorders. The incidence of anorexia nervosa runs as high as seven percent in professional dance schools in North America and Europe. The incidence of bulimia is more difficult to determine, because bulimia does not usually produce emaciation, and the symptoms are therefore more easily kept secret (1985).

Politics

Politics exists in the dance world as in any other. Students or performers may be the butt of bias, victim of favoritism, "defendant" of disloyalty, or object of intrigue by someone's self-aggrandize-ment. These situations may create stress. An individual who feels mistreated might seek a neutral person to help assess the situation, make suggestions, or try to remedy the stressor.

Improvisation Movement and Contemplative Creativity

Dissatisfaction with elements of the dance styles and their re-lated training and professional practices of a particular time often catalyze new movements and genres. For example, unhappiness with the structure of the ballet world and what it represents, its male dominance, traditional movement dictates, training require-ments, choreography, performance, and production provoked the "modern" dance rebellion of Isadora Duncan, Loie Fuller, and suc-cessive generations of modern dancers. Modern dance in turn evoked the genre generally labelled postmodern dance.

Dance improvisation, referring to movements or choreographic decisions not fully set before they are performed, may be viewed as a reaction to the three above-mentioned dance genres. Improvisa-tion participation may be a way to resist and reduce the stress of hi-erarchical teacher-student relationships, being collectively molded to an authoritative ideal of a particular dance style, and the strati-fied performance star system.

According to a survey of about 150 people from the United States and Canada, the improvisation movement's egalitarian na-ture and allowance for individuality, a strong tradition beginning with modern dance, attracted participants (Novack, 1984). Some appreciate the noncompetitive atmosphere in which individuals "play with one another," a contrast with the usual pattern of stu-dent competition for teacher attention and approval. Improvisa-tion is a way of "shaking loose from set movement patterns and erasing some of the 'imprints of traditional dance technique'" as well as differentiating oneself from a teacher or a tradition (p. 2).

Moreover, the improviser engaging in an activity requiring com-munal group experience of unpredictable cooperative and egalitar-ian interactions allows the experience of self-awareness and self-discovery as a person and not just as a dancer. In this sense, improvisation has elements of dance therapy. Improvisers thus see dance as a transforming experience. The audience can identify with the process of the dancer's immediate decision-making and creativity.

Improvisation is a prominent practice at the Dance/Movement Studies Department of the Naropa Institute in Boulder, Colorado. Here it is combined with "sitting contemplation" and contemplative choreography. The concern has been on presenting dance/movement from a contemplative point of view.

"Sitting meditation" is about "coming to stillness" and ultimately "connecting directly with the raw energy of the phenomenal world. The state of mind cultivated by sitting practice is open, inquisitive and clear, thus enabling a person to produce art that relates more directly and genuinely with one's experience" (Rockwell, 1988). Naropa philosophy and practice derive from the Buddhist tradition of *shamatha/vipashyana*, or mindfulness/awareness practice. On the one hand, *shamatha* trains the individual through the development of a synchronicity of body, speech, and mind in order to focus personal experience on a moment-to-moment awareness without the distractions of past or future. On the other hand, *vipashyana*, developing out of the mindfulness practice, provides a more panoramic or broader vision of the environment. An attempt is made to become calm and detached from habitual ways of perceiving based on the entrapment of "ego" or a self-centered way of existence.

Barbara Dilley, a former performer with the Merce Cunningham Company, Judson Dance Theatre, and Grand Union in New York City says,

> I was interested in what it would be like for other dancers to slow down and work with training their minds. I wanted to help them peel away the unnecessary aspects of their training and become more basic, more fundamental. It is not that I wanted to throw out the American dance tradition. It seems there is an aspect of the American creative process that is genuine and clear; but then there is another aspect that is highly neurotic, escapist, and fun-

damentally aggressive. I wanted to start at the beginning, and then sort it out from there (quoted in Pierpoint, 1984).

Economic Survival

"Consider this for the classifieds: Wanted—Able-Bodied, athletic, esthetically sensitive type for short career in the arts. Approximately 10 years' training and apprenticeship required. Must perform well under pressure while injured or ill. High threshold of pain necessary. Must tolerate verbal abuse and ridicule. Minimum nine hours per day. Weekends. Travel four months of the year. Artistic satisfaction. $12,000 to $17,000 per year." Ron Reagan, son of the president of the United States thus began his explanation of why he quit the ballet (1983). He pointed out that dancers are "willing slaves to an art in which management calls the shots and holds their contracts."

Performing artists are more prone to unemployment than other members of the workforce. A 1980 study, *Employment in the Performing Arts: Reality and Myth*, by the Labor Institute for Human Enrichment, found 76 percent of the professional dancers experienced some unemployment compared with 18 percent for other members of the workforce (*Washington Post*, 1983). And because dance offers seasonal rather than full-time work, not having enough weeks of performance to be eligible for unemployment insurance is a powerful stressor.

Dancers usually operate without the security of standardized, union-approved contracts. Freelance artists can rarely strike effectively. They are easily and quickly replaced. Not only do American dancers receive little income, but most lack health insurance and are neither on salary nor pension to which they would be entitled if they pursued a number of years in the career.

Even in one of the foremost ballet companies in the world, where dancers have steady jobs and are among the highest paid, economic survival is a problem. Bentley says about money: "I really think we are the most ignorant paid people on earth. I'm sure we are constantly cheated and never complain. Money is only to pay for the apartment, to buy a fur coat and ballet clothes" (1982), p. 18). Principal dancers in New York may dole out 40 to 50 percent of their income for rent alone. Kirkland remarked, "The routine of daily practice and preparation kept me shuttling in taxis all day. In addition to classes and rehearsals at various studios in the city, I regularly visited health clubs for swimming, whirlpool treatments, and sauna, and more specialized facilities for massage and physical therapy. The expenses added up, so that I was always broke. Whatever discretionary dollars remained in my personal budget went into practice clothes, wigs, cosmetics, and a myriad of related items, including costumes whenever the need arose" (1986, p. 185).

Conflicting interests create stress. For example, in 1980 the dancers at New York City Ballet and management had come to a deadlock and a strike seemed imminent. Mr. B., as the dancers lovingly addressed Balanchine, was told and was predictably upset and emotional. He said he would do his best, and if the dancers wanted to run the company, he would leave with his ballets. "Oh God, how awful we feel; we only want enough money to pay the rent. Many of the younger kids simply cannot afford it. Their parents have to help them. Mr. B. takes it personally, of course, We are his company, his creation, his tools; without him we are nothing, and without us—well, he needs us, but he can always find dancers. The question seems rather basic: do we want to fight for our own pockets, or do we give a little for him? We . . . love him. We will show him that—and maybe scrimp a little more" (Bentley, 1982,p. 64–65).

"Mr. Balanchine is our leader, our president, our mother, our father, our friend, our guide, our mentor, our destiny. He knows all, sees all, and controls all—all of us. . . . We are all his children" (p. 58–59). Bentley observed, "They say he has always dictated and had his own way with us, and we will stand for it no longer" (p. 87). Yet those who love themselves more than Balanchine, many of whom barely know him since the company has grown so large, made their stand. "They cry they have belief in him as an artist but not as their dictator. But how can one separate the two when his art can be produced only out of a state that he alone must rule? It's a pity he needs a hundred individuals as his tools rather than paint-brushes" (p. 89).

A key issue of economic survival is the conflict between needing to raise money from the public or private sector and maintaining artistic integrity in addition to time to create. Most dance groups depend on grants to survive, since the arts rarely pay for themselves. Arts councils could not easily give money directly to artists to create new works, so dancers spend time and money to form tax-free educational foundations. Then the question arises as to who owns the creative work.

National state and local arts agencies use peer review for dance funding proposals. A problem arises when evaluators favor a particular style at a specific point in time. This may induce some conformity and compromise of aesthetic goals. To obtain government grants, one usually needs favorable reviews from critics, and they, too, have their biases. Moreover, an art agency grant often provides the imprimateur necessary for private funding.

Economic pressures turn dance into a business. Grants often require work to be produced in certain seasons for fiscal reasons. Companies may not develop new works because administrators prefer known box office quantities.

When there is economic constriction, the arts are the first to experience cutbacks. "The less money there is available, the higher the degree of selling," said Present Company's artistic director, Wendy Woodson. "Right now we are in an era of: How much can we play up to the bourgeois establishment and get money from them" (quoted in McIntyre, 1986). She thinks there is too much business now in art, because "there is a point at which they are incompatible. It's a very delicate balance—if you are too much into making money, the purpose of doing art is diminished."

What keeps Woodson and her collaborator Achim Nowak focused on that artistic purpose is their work at community-oriented institutions. Of course, audience expectation and innovative choreography may create economic crises. Groups have to give the audience what it wants in order to attract spectators. At the same time, dancers try to stretch and brainwash the audience to accept new images.

In many parts of the United States, finding low-cost space for dance studios, rehearsal, and performance can be stressful. The problem of real estate needs for the dance profession and other arts organizations has gotten so severe that the New York City Department of Cultural Affairs and Office of Business Development commissioned a study of spaces for the arts within its jurisdiction (Alliance for the Arts, 1985). There is a severe shortage of affordable, appropriate space in the areas of Manhattan that have served for many years as centers of arts activity. Until recently, there was inexpensive, suitable real estate in abundant supply in the "valley" between the high-rise areas of Lower Manhattan and Midtown Manhattan. As older, commercial and industrial structures in areas like SoHo, Tribeca, NoHo, and Chelsea lost their traditional tenants, substantial space was leased to arts organizations at low rates. Then rising rents in Midtown and Lower Manhattan caused many commercial tenants to relocate to the "valley" and push up rents as much as 200 to 300 percent. Between 1985 and 1987, in an area between 56th and 92nd Streets, west of Avenue of the Americas, 55 studio spaces were eliminated (Dunning, 1987). Since small dance groups have performance seasons of a few weeks at most, performance spaces are shared. But with only a small number of these dance performance spaces, each serving many companies, their continued existence is critical.

Because New York City is the dance capital of the world, soloists and companies need to perform there for the *imprimatur* of the New York City dance critics (Hanna, 1985). Yet, the costs are often prohibitive. The Alwin Nikolais Company has complicated lighting and its own technician, yet, because of union regulations, a theater house technician must be paid anyway.

Touring is a necessity for many dance groups to survive, since they only support a short season in most home locales. But touring, with the need to sublet one's apartment, jet lag, new foods, abrupt climatic changes, different kinds of stages, and disruption of social relationships, is stressful. Often facilities are inadequate and conducive to injury. New York City Ballet had refused to perform at the Kennedy Center for the Performing Arts in Washington, D.C. until it changed its floor.

Some ballet companies struggling to control costs have taken up twin residencies. At least 10 companies have second home arrangements. For example, the Joffrey Ballet based in New York City has a second home in Los Angeles; Cincinnati Ballet, in New Orleans; Washington Ballet in Baltimore; Don Wagoner and Dancers in New York and South Carolina; Cleveland Ballet, in San Jose; Pilobolus Dance Theatre in Washington and Connecticut; Merce Cunningham in New York and Minnesota; and Pittsburg Ballet Theatre, in Savanna.

Commentary

Given society's attitude toward dancers, the choreographer and dance company treatment of dancers, the brevity of a performing career, the hazards of injury, the low financial rewards (except for a few superstars), and the economics of the dance process, production, and performance, a person who pursues the dance career with all its stressors is a unique individual. Passion for the dance is a key motivation. Some individuals seek out dance as an occupation because of its challenges and their psychological needs; the competition pushes them to greater achievements. They become accustomed to the pressures and learn how to manage the effects of stress in a constructive manner. Stress has spurred the development of new dance forms and stress management techniques. Some dancers, however, resort to self-pernicious measures of coping with stress such as improper eating, drug abuse, and performing with injuries. Still others choose to change careers. Efforts have been made in the dance world to alter the public perception of the performance career and to improve the working conditions of the occupation itself to make it more like mainstream jobs with contracts, insurance, salaries, and pensions.

Chapter 10
Resisting, Reducing, and Escaping Stress in Western Amateur Dancing

Amateur dancing occurs in private and public social settings, from homes to churches, schools to nightclubs, and in dance classes at studios, schools, and community centers. Even though amateurs rarely dance in a theater for an audience, they are often cognizant of and affected by others watching them in social or dance class settings. Thus amateur dancers may experience the kind of performance anxiety described for professional dancers. Moreover, amateurs may be stressed by feelings of awkwardness and social incompetence when they are unable to make their feet do what the mind's eye wants them to do.

Dancing Madness, Rock, and Disco

Social dances such as rock or disco are most often a flow activity that help an individual to resist stress through developing physical fitness and to escape stress through immersion in the dance. The music feeds and energizes dancers who then emanate energy contagiously to invigorate other people in the dance setting. There may be a mass elation, a communitas or merging with the crowd. Dancers can communicate and interact with others, using their bodies in ways that are not done in everyday life. By focusing on a limited stimulus field, dancers lose the self or feel in control of the self or a social situation. Dancers offered these comments: "Once I get into it, then I just float along, having fun, just feeling myself move around," "I get sort of a physical high from it . . . very sweaty, very feverish or sort of ecstatic when everything is going really well" (Hendin and Csikszentmihalyi, pp. 104–105).

Stress may be induced when dancers get insufficient feedback in this improvisational, rather than choreographically set, activity to know whether they are doing well or poorly. Furthermore, response from one's partner may be ambiguous. Determining whether movements are a sexual advance or merely a dance pattern is often difficult. A male explained, "You can always say you were dancing and not flirting. So you can do all kinds of things, and then act like, 'That was the way it went,' or if you get picked up, fine" (ibid.). Some people felt self-conscious, embarrassed, or threatened because of the bystanders.

Social dances often offer an opportunity for adolescents and young adults to release, with society's sanction, a variety of strong feelings which under most other circumstances they are required to suppress or repress. Each generation has its own movements, along with dress codes and music, to set itself apart, to create a sense of belonging to the "group," and to respond to its own social milieu and earlier styles. Of course, social dances permit interpersonal relations and finding sexual partners. Dancing is part of the rite of passage and courtship toward adulthood.

The turn-of-the-century New York City working-class young women escaped to the dance halls (Peiss, 1986). Dancing alleviated the tedium of work as well as permitted the expression of sexuality in ragtime movements (the waltz, spieling, tough dancing, slow rag, lover's two-step, turkey trot, grizzly bear, and bunny hop) that would have been unacceptable in any other public manner. The dance setting was a place to go to get away from a disliked job or nagging family. There were stresses related to sexuality:

> Working-class women received conflicting messages about the virtues of virginity in their daily lives. Injunctions about chastity from parents, church, and school might conflict with the lived experience of urban labor and leisure. Working in factories and stores often entailed forms of sexual harassment that instructed

women to exchange sexual favors for economic gain, while talk about dates and sexual exploits helped to pass the working day. Crowded tenement homes caused working-class daughters to pursue their social life in the unprotected spaces of the streets, while those living in boarding homes contended with the attentions of male lodgers. The pleasure and freedom young women craved could be found in the social world of dance halls, but these also carried a mixed message, permitting expressive female sexuality within a context of dependency and vulnerability (p. 110).

The dance gave the women a new-found sense of freedom at the same time the men had the prerogatives of selecting partners and breaking in on dancers. Moreover, women relied on men's treats to see them through the evening's entertainment.

In the mid 1960s girls liked speeded-up dances; boys, the unhurried ones (Blum, 1966–67). The comments of the adolescents reveal dance as escape from stress and dissipation of tension: "The more we frug, the more South Vietnam, lung cancer, and getting into your father's college fade into the distance" (p. 359); "The dances offer temporary retreat from a complex environment with which youth seems to feel inadequately equipped to cope" (p. 362); "The feeling is of complete thoughtlessness. The Buddhists would have called it Nirvana," (p. 359); "It exhausts any built up strength [tension] due to anger or anxiety" (p. 360).

Since the disco dance delirium of the 1970s, partners in many settings move as they please, independently and in unison. Revelers participate in a state of liminality at which time social class and organizational barriers temporarily dissolve as people partake of the inverse of the bureaucratic normal world of work. The social order is rearranged on the weekend, and the week's tension is dissipated. For some people, living in a world where work and dance are so bifurcated conduces to stress.

As is the case for professional dance, display of the instrument of dance, the body, in the amateur dance context may enhance the dancer's self-image and thus resist or reduce stress. Students who took folk dance classes, when compared with those who did not take classes, were more positive about their self-concept and body concept (Silver, 1981).

Marathons

From about 1910 on, as part of a dance craze that swept the United States, social dance fads have cascaded into the popular consciousness. These dances fulfill the same dance-stress functions as the recent rock dance or the much earlier "tarantism." The marathon, a special case of "besotted performance" that occurred during the depression, coincided with changing social and cultural patterns, including heterosexual relationships (Martin, 1986). The dance was called the latest form of St. Vitus Dance (Calabria, 1976, p. 57).

Non-stop marathons offered the dancers material respite from the stress of poverty as well as catharsis and temporary escape. The marathons offered the audience empathic catharsis and divertissement from this problems. Promoters made money.

Advertisements over the radio and in the papers solicited contestants. The endurance dancing of marathons attracted unemployed youth with nothing to do who were willing to suffer for the dream of a payoff, winning prize money for survival. There would usually be $1000, a good amount at the time, divided up: $600 went to the winning couple, and the last prize was $50. In addition, spectators threw money at their favorite dancers. Besides, the dancers received food and medical attention; often there was a trainer, nurse, and judge on each 12-hour shift. George Eells, an enthusiastic audience member at countless marathons during his youth, remarked, "There was a strong personality type that was attracted to this kind of thing. I think they would've adjusted just as well to being in jail or being in the army. . . .the promoter took care of them and helped them make decisions. He got them out of jail when they were in jail; he helped them if they got into a financial bind. And then he took advantage of them and made lots of money off of them" (quoted in Martin, p. 16).

The immediacy of the marathon appealed to the audience. Every kind of person came: High school students and old ladies with their knitting, wealthy oil people who thought they were slumming, and people from the sports world, red light district, and middle class. The spectators could identify with the suffering the dancers projected; it made them feel better about their own problems. Some contests deteriorated into physical brutality. A former onlooker said, "I remember feeling slightly guilty about enjoying somebody else's suffering. It seemed sadistic in away" (p. 14). Another oldtimer said, "Now, people came to see 'em die. That's an over-statement. But they came to see 'em suffer, and to see when they were going to fall down. They wanted to see if their favorites were going to make it. That was all part of it. It was Depression entertainment" (p. 7).

Some marathoners became professionals and married, divorced, and married again as they not only danced but conducted the routines of their daily lives in public while keeping in rhythm. Lives were in turmoil." It was a heightening of what you find in ordinary society because it was all enclosed in one room," said Eells (quoted in Martin, p. 17).

Slam Dancing

The 1980s witnessed a new dance genre in New York City and Los Angeles. Slam dancing, with a scary surface, was perhaps a way for adolescent males to deal with the stressors of maturation, aggressive personal feelings, and violence in the society at large. Through dancing the youths achieve euphoria, enhanced self-concept, and a healthy fatigue.

This is a scene from the A7 club on the Lower East Side (Sommer, 1983): The crowd, 85 percent male, white and under 20, whether hardcore musicians, dancers or onlookers, dresses alike in "black combat boots, old Levis and black belts, almost-white T-shirts or flannel plaids, and shaved heads" (p. 29). The youths, mostly middle-class and suburban, travel to Manhattan's tough neighborhoods to "dance dangerously and look malevolent" (p. 31)).

The male dancers, after standing about staring at the singer, erupt on the dance floor.

Heads down, bodies hunkered over, arms flailing, they pound across the floor slamming into each other, the wall, and the watchers. Staggering in get-down fighting position, they lift up their knees, sometimes doing a spastic cross-over step, crashing each boot down. They slam into flesh and plaster, crash off-balance, and are immediately pulled up and pushed back into the tumult. They scramble on top of each other's shoulders, "chicken-slamming," thwacking together, crunching to the floor in "pile-ons." Now they move into a rough circle "thrashing," elbows out, arms propellers, stomping and hopping like speeding Indians at a nightmare pow-wow. Faces grimace, eyebrows draw together (p. 29).

The males celebrate "raw power and barely contained fury." They are ecstatic. As they run amok, they are still within safety. "This activity is about support (chicken-slams, help-ups and push backs) and cooperation (circle thrash). The crowd is a willing pillow. If it were really vicious, people would simply step aside and let divers go splat. Or they could kick the shit out of floored dancers (ibid.). This is not to say that there are no injuries. As with any sport, injuries are endured as symbols of macho courage.

Folk Dancing

Amateur folk dancing allows people to cope with stress in a variety of ways, including escaping from technological society and returning to human contact. One dancer explained: "Folk dancing keeps things on a human plane. . . . Part of the etiquette of contra dancing is the eye contact." Another said, "It's great for business travel. You get to a new town, call someone from the folk dance network and spend the evening dancing. There's no other social activity in which you touch someone the same evening you meet them."

Yet another man agrees: "Where else can you spend $4 and put your hands on a hundred women?" (McNees, 1987).

The Ballroom Dance Studio

"'Exposes' by information media, lawsuits by allegedly victimized persons and negative side smiles by society at large" reveal stressors for students and teachers active in the United States ballroom dance studio business of providing adults with the skills utilized in the "polite companionship" of social dancing (Lopata and Noel, 1972). The studios attract defenseless, lonely people who want primary relations with the opposite sex—affection, trust, reciprocity, and concern with mutual feelings—so badly that they are willing to use studios to buy them. The studio puts on regular or special event "parties" that duplicate social occasions on the outside. Students, teachers, and teacher trainees are encouraged to bring guests to the studio to witness lessons or attend the parties, for guests are an important source of new students.

Students experience stress to the extent that the dance activities are neither the means to develop social skills of moving, talking, and dressing nor to acquire social relationships with the teachers and other students after substantial monetary expenditures. Upon discovering the actual cost for the services, students are often shocked. In the early 1970s "lessons at chain schools cost between $5 and $9 per half-hour or $10 to $18 for the standard one hour. Thus an introductory course of 30 hours costs the student anywhere between $300 and $540. Most studios attempt to enroll students for at least 100 hours for $1,000–$1,800 but, as several well-publicized lawsuits have pointed out, women have been known to sign up for lessons totaling more than $10,000" (pp. 188–89).

Management pressures the teachers not only to teach the students to dance, but to sign them up for "renewals" for large blocks of lessons or even for life-time courses.

A Ballet Dance Class

Physical fitness and escape from everyday stresses are the bounty of the dance class for some students. Linda Valleroy observed herself and other ballet hobbyists:

Up the stairs in your business clothes. You hear the piano playing Chopin. You are beat, but suddenly begin to feel a little happier. Into the practice clothes, the shoes. You talk to some girlfriends about how the Kirov is coming to town. Already you are feeling a lot happier and then class starts. Concentrate. Keep the flow of energy moving. Don't sit in the plies. Pull up the knees. Oops, there goes that stupid tension in my arm, again. How can I ever keep my pelvis parallel in *rond de jambes*? God, they are hard. They have always been hard. This is the litany of the anatomy.

Now, after all these years of ballet I am starting on a new system. I play anatomy class at the *barre* and really try to dance in the center. Sometimes I really dance. But you know, it's a few seconds here, a few seconds there. Anyway, by the end of class I am generally always so happy. The others are happy, too. You just have to close your eyes and listen to the voice quality in the dressing room. People talk faster. Their voices are high pitched. And, I keep wondering what did it. What was it that made the world seem like an enchanting place, again? Whatever it was is what keeps me paying my seven dollars there as opposed to some wine bar (personal communication, 1986).

Valleroy reflected upon what seemed to create the state of euphoria. There are several interrelated factors. Because one focuses on a complicated set of anatomical maneuvers, all the body placement positions, the flow of energy and the quality of the movement, and tempo of the music, there is no time to think about one's identity and problems. The individual mentally and physically realigns the body, because ballet is a unique postural system that requires an uplifting posture. Mastery over the body and greater physical fitness leads to self-confidence. So does enlarging one's social network. Class is planned continuous movement which lasts an hour or more, and endorphin levels are highest in exercise over an hour. Valleroy thinks the ballet dance class is a "regression to a childhood state, far, far, from the adult professional world. Many women in adult ballet classes are career women who struggle with adult [and feminine] problems in a man's world during the [play-less work] day. At night you can be a little kid again, or a swan, or a princess. These mental images will not get one very far in the work world. What a relief to be a swan."

Aerobic Dance

Aerobic dance, as described in the second chapter, has potential for physical and psychological benefits. This genre combines simple dance steps and locomotor patterns. Evidence of psychological benefits comes from a study of female teachers who participated in an aerobic dance program in an educational employment setting. The teachers showed decreased symptoms of burnout and improved relations among teacher colleagues as well as between themselves and administrators. Moreover, the teachers' students found their teachers to be more knowledgeable, poised, lively, and interesting (Forman, 1983).

Dancing and Relaxation Exercises

Senior citizens involved in dancing and relaxation exercises manifested benefits that nonparticipants did not. The dancers had a slower heart rate (Holcomb, 1977).

Commentary

Individuals participate in social dancing or dance classes for pleasure, exercise, marking self-identity, and meeting people. The dance may help to resist stress through developing physical fitness and building social support that extends beyond the dance setting. Reduction of stress may occur through the dissipation of quotidian tensions of work and family as well as crises such as depression or war. Escape from stress occurs through the flow and ecstasy of multisensory envelopment or the fantasy and enchantment of a romantic dance genre. Amateur dance may induce stress through performance anxiety, insufficient social dance invitations or dance class support from teacher or classmates, and ambiguous performance feedback.

Chapter 11
Receiving Dance (Movement) Therapy Vis-à-vis Stress

Purposes and Approaches

✗ Dance therapy is the Western psychotherapeutic use of movement in a process that furthers the physical, emotional, and cognitive integration of an individual. The process acknowledges the fusion of mind and body and the expressive and communicative primacy of nonverbal body movement in revealing aspects of a person's state of mind, personality, and range of adaptive behaviors. The notion that movement patterns may support or contradict verbal behavior is recognized. So, too, is the premise that people may be able to express themselves and communicate better through nonverbal than verbal means. There is an assumption that individual growth and well-being depend on self-expression and communication of feelings.

A dance therapist assists a person to work through problems in order to gain insight, change behavior, establish emotional contact with other humans, and release tension. Dance/movement therapy may be an integral component of a broad treatment program or a primary intervention.

Therapists observe an individual's or family's movements for diagnostic purposes, treatment goals, and assessment of change over time as a result of therapy (see *American Journal of Dance Therapy*; Mason, 1974; Delaney, 1982; Bernstein, 1979; and Levanthal, 1983). Practitioners read a patient's/client's posture, gesture, face, use of space (distance between people), synchrony with others, manner of touch, and eye gaze. Training in dancer Rudolf Laban's methods of analyzing and symbolically representing dynamic and spatial aspects of movement (as developed by his disciples) helps in observing and recording movement in the process of a dance therapy session. Research seeks movement parameters indicative of suicidal risk and other less severe stress responses.

Certified dance therapists as well as psychologists, psychiatrists, counselors, social workers, and sensitivity trainers may use dance or movement in therapy. Many practitioners consider specific ritual dances, such as the ones that have been described in earlier chapters, to be the genesis of the therapeutic use of dance in the West.

It is noteworthy that the term "stress" is not as common in the literature of dance therapy as other concepts that can be subsumed under stress. Dance therapy is used to help individuals to overcome and resist stress-related problems. The therapeutic process is especially helpful to people who have difficulty in verbalization.

Dance therapy does not use a standard dance form or movement technique. Any genre, from African folk to European waltz, may be drawn upon. Improvisation is common. Much of what is called dance therapy does not appear to be what we usually call dance but rather movement or predance warm-up type exercises. A therapist may match another person's muscle tension changes and adopt the same body shape. Some therapists use *ideokinesis*, having clients image sensory awareness in order to relax overtense muscles. Numerous therapists draw upon Alexander or Jacobson techniques, Dalcroze rhythmic methods, yoga striving for inner peace, and Dervish turning to achieve altered states of consciousness. Many therapists attempt to have clients alleviate tension to facilitate the flow of expression by making use of the full range of movement qualities that have been described by Laban and his followers. Issues of dependency, fight/flight, and pairing come to the fore.

The reason for such variety lies in the broad spectrum of populations that undergo dance therapy: for example, self-actualizers (individuals who cope well with daily life but desire to be more in touch with their expressive body actions), neurotic, psychotic, retarded, sociopathic (e.g., delinquent, battered women, drug addicts), physically handicapped, and geriatric. Dance therapists may work with staff in a mental health setting to sensitize them to their own movement behavior and the movement of patients so that staff behavior becomes more effective in interaction with patients. Some therapists prefer the term "dance" to "movement" because the former implies stereotypic joy and well-being. Moreover dance therapy certification requires many years of dance training.

The condition of a client/patient in dance therapy varies from being under acute or chronic traumatic stress to experiencing minor stress. Therapists may treat severely disturbed patients in the back wards of psychiatric hospitals and other long-term institutions, and other clients in community health centers, nursing homes, private practice offices, clinics, special educational settings, and the client's home.

Dance therapy underpinning may come from the human potential, holistic health, or medical models. The humanistic and holistic health approaches have in common the belief that individuals share responsibility for their therapeutic progress and relationships with others. By contrast, the medical model assumes that the therapist is responsible for treatment and cure.

There are various, but not usually mutually exclusive, theoretical approaches to dance therapy that do not necessarily require different physical techniques (Bernstein, 1979). Dance therapy is grounded in the worlds of dance and psychology. Some dance therapy approaches, such as Marian Chace's pioneering work, derive from experimentation with dance; other approaches derive from psychoanalysis or are aligned with behavior modification. The majority of therapists ascribe to one or more theoretical frames of reference such as the following:

Psychoanalysis, developed by Sigmund Freud, offers dance therapy a diagnostic tool in its theory of stages of physical and psychological maturation. The *Freudian* developmental theory assumes that through therapy the client outgrows an inefficient, fixated, or infantile mode and dissolves resistances. A vital concept is *transference:* people become emotionally engaged with the therapist as a stand in for a significant figure out of the past. (In therapy the psychological moment in a person's life when he or she suffered hurts may be recreated so that the person may see how this was experienced and thus gain insights for improved functioning.) The individual's make-up, conflicts, and defenses manifest themselves in the dance process which is seen as a symbolic reflection of the psychological state of the individual and a vehicle to a new state. Freud emphasized the body as the basis of the ego, the part of the self that mediates between inner strivings and outer demands. Motility is, therefore, part of the ego apparatus (Siegel, E., 1984). Dance therapy helps to release and sublimate repressed psychosexual and aggressive impulses. Within the psychoanalytic field, the work of Wilhelm Reich, C. Gustav Jung, and Henry Stack Sullivan, among others, guides dance therapy.

Reich was concerned not only with what a patient said, but how the person moved. He believed that the walk, stance, and breath patterns revealed a specific character type. Reich thought chronic muscular tension indicated repression and blocked the expression of affect. Illustrative is the holding of the chest area as a sign of repressed feelings of need and longing. Dance therapy attempts to reduce muscular tension, what Reich calls the "defensive armor," to facilitate regained mobility.

Within the *Jungian* approach, dance is an expression of healing rather than a projection of personality or psychopathology and evidence of disease and disorder. Art is considered the means by which patients may objectify themselves. Participation in dance therapy evokes conscious and unconscious fantasies and conflicts that are available for analysis and catharsis.

Sullivan's *interpersonal theory of personality* holds that the individual develops through the accumulated experience of self in interaction with others. The experience, or perception of the interaction rather than its objectivity, is what matters in this process. Therapists following Sullivan attempt to resocialize the individual's interpersonal style with other people in order to develop more successful nonstressful social relationships.

Learning theory considers dance as a basic need and a safe insulated arena through which to explore feelings and thoughts in order to renew old values or introduce new ones and thereby change behavior. The orientation of *communication theory* is that different ways of expression and communication may be blocked, congruent, or conflicting. Mediated by dance, insights facilitate verbal reflexivity and resolution of conflicting messages. The *cognitive behavior approach* seeks through dance to reverse faulty thinking patterns and negative feelings about the self.

Gestalt-phenomenological theory emphasizes "awareness, excitement, and involvement (responsibility and contact) in the moment-to-moment process of living" (Serlin, 1977, p. 145). This approach precludes the therapist's predetermined judgment and prestructure. Spontaneously responding to a new situation, a dance-therapist helps someone acquire self-knowledge and acceptance in order to grow.

Psychomotor developmental theory posits that individuals who have difficulty adapting can improve their lives by recouping those movement components usually experienced in the normal growth process. The *pragmatic approach* assumes that a dance therapist should be able to deal with any kind of situation, since other modes of therapy may be unavailable. Practitioners with this orientation draw upon whatever theory and method seems most applicable to the client's condition.

The pattern of interpersonal relations varies in dance therapy sessions. Therapy may take place solely in a dyadic therapist/client interaction, with a family, or in a group that includes the therapist and several or more clients. Interpersonal dancing is designed to enhance empathy and trust between individuals. A group dancing together is potentially nurturing for some clients.

On the basis of *group therapy theory* and clinical experience, Schmais offers a preliminary categorization of eight interrelated healing processes in guided group dance therapy (1985). These processes operate in many of the ritual, social, and theatrical dances mentioned earlier. (1) Synchrony refers to people moving together, in time or making the same spatial design with the same body parts, or effort, irrespective of body parts. Movement synchrony is often supported by touch, visual contact, and/or sounds and words toward promoting group solidarity, resocialization, and expression.

(2) Expression as a goal is predicated on the notion that external-ization of internal states makes them less ominous, especially in a group setting that provides a supportive matrix for shameful and frightening feelings. (3) Rhythm serves to integrate, inspire, and regulate the dance therapy participation process. (4) Vitalization, investing people with the power to live, occurs through moving. "The flow of motion connects limbs to torso and feelings to ac-tions. . . . In the dance therapy session there is a synergistic effect resulting from the stimulation of being in a group situation and from the activation that is caused by moving" (p. 25).

(5) Integration in dance therapy describes the dynamic accom-plishment of a sense of unity within the individual and a sense of community between internal and external reality. "For most pa-tients, the accretive process begins with a simple motion, perhaps a flick of the wrist. The therapist repeats the movement, adding de-scriptive phrases and poetic images to enhance the meaning and crystallize the action. As the energy level rises, the gesture of a sin-gle joint can become a postural motion spreading through the en-tire body, cutting through tension and engaging inert areas. The facial expressions, sounds and words become congruent with the body actions. Body parts connect, discordant rhythms disappear and distracting gestures dissolve" (pp. 27–28).

(6) Cohesion refers to the social bond that exists in dance content and form. Steps toward people actively participating in each oth-er's symbolic statements include the group connecting through the rhythmic beat, auditory and visual feedback from members of the group, physical closeness, and touching, first of oneself to experi-ence self-awareness and then of others such as in a light tapping of another's shoulder or hand. "As they dance out each person's pri-vate story, the story teller finds acceptance and sees himself as ac-ceptable. Barriers of isolation dissolve, and people feel that they can once again enter a social world" (p. 31).

(7) Education refers to clients/patients learning from their own experiences as well as from others, especially through participating in others' symbolic expressions. "For example, when a patient mir-rors someone else dancing out a theme of sorrow, he may encoun-ter his own unfinished mourning, he may learn about the many

ways people deal with loss and he may become aware of the necessity of accepting the inevitability of death. . . . As the group affect
escalates, patients see others change and realize that they too are
changing, and that change is possible. . . . Coming to the sessions
with anxiety, annoyance and little enthusiasm, patients learn that
the act of moving itself can reduce tensions, diminish depression
and increase energy. . . . By being trusted to support someone else
or to lead the group, they learn to trust themselves and to take initiative. And when powerful feelings are exposed as part of the
dance, patients learn that expressing emotions does not necessarily
lead to disaster" (pp. 31–32).

(8) Symbolism is "probably the least understood and most valuable process in dance therapy" (p. 33). It requires a certain technical
mastery to abstract and structure what is seen, felt, and imag-
ined. . . . Symbolic expressions in dance therapy form the bridge
between the patient's internal and external worlds as they transfer
energy from one realm to the other in a social context" to allow for
psychic distance from private preoccupations (pp. 33–34).

Akstein (1973) capitalized on possession states described in
Chapter 3 to develop a new type of group psychotherapy: *Terpsichoreotrancetherapy* (TTT). Analogous to the Brazilian sects, trance
is supported by music from the Umbanda sect and is performed in
a theatrical setting. The TTT, however, discards the mystic. Members of the social class to which the patient is accustomed comprise
the therapy group. TTT technique bears some resemblance to hypnosis. Although a director gives instructions for patients to close
their eyes, concentrate on one thing they wish to accomplish to increase their rate of breathing (hyperventilation), no other oral communication with patients occurs. Every patient has an assistant
nearby on the alert against falls. Patients may dance the samba,
sway, or burst into violent trance. Those who develop a deep
trance, dance slowly, and display a tranquil countenance achieve a
sense of well-being after the session. The calmness gives the patient the means to better face and solve problems.

Therapy based on *Eastern Buddist philosophy*, such as the human
potential model at the Naropa Institute discussed in Chapter 9,
aims to wake up and to uplift people. The artistic process is seen as

part of everyday life. "The implications of this are that everyone is an artist and that we are always making art or that there is no distinction between art and anything else you do" (Rockwell, 1988).

Illustrative Stress Situations and Dance Therapy

Americans *migrating* to rural areas in order to escape the stresses of city living may find adjusting to the different country problems difficult. They may feel alienation from established residents, the isolation of country living, the lack of jobs, and winter cabin fever. Dance is among the useful therapeutic coping techniques (*Behavioral Medicine*, 1979).

There is no question that *aging* brings new stress to one's life. And the increasing American population of elderly people faces loneliness, insecurity, depression, confusion, anxiety, and anger. Lerman (1984) addresses the benefits and approaches to dance for senior citizens.

Schoenfeld leads dance therapy groups in nursing groups, a vehicle for "patients to escape the limitations of their disabilities, sicknesses, and restrictions. Although dealing on a primary level with the limitations of the physical self, the space around that self, and the emotions, my patients can escape these limitations through dance. . . . Expression, exercise, catharsis, group recognition, and acceptance are all important goals in the sessions, but I think the rediscovery of the joy of moving in a creative and aesthetic sense has been the greatest reward for their hard efforts" (1986).

She knows she cannot erase the realities of institutional living nor extensively treat individual psychological problems: "What I can do is facilitate a sense of self-worth within each participant despite the necessary compromises in mobility, focus, sightedness, comprehension, and ability to verbalize."

A typical session involves the following: "Gentle stretching and deep breathing, usually unaccompanied by music, start the class. Arms are moved upward, downward, out to the sides, forward, back, and in circles. Every part of the body is moved—hips are wiggled, knees are lifted, legs are carefully stretched. A beachball helps in the process. We join in unison clapping, even if only one hand can be used, in differing rhythms. Music in a variety of moods lends energy, stimulates, and calms.

"Choreographically, we move around in a circle, pairing up, mirroring each other's movements, sometimes emulating a little performance with a soloist in the center of the circle. Sometimes we create a congaline formation with the mobile greeting those seated—everyone getting into the act. The patients end the class dancing to the elevators, and I wish them a good lunch."

Sandel worked among nursing home residents where the longing for companionship, fear of physical deterioration, and sexual frustration commonly emerged in movement therapy sessions. She found that sound and movement activities create an atmosphere of excitement that revitalize geriatric patients. Moreover, the therapist may be the first recipient of clients' erotic fantasies. Sexually provocative behavior toward the therapist, she said, may mask feelings of neediness or rage. The therapist can use individual transferences to facilitate the development of a group identity and peer interaction.

Among many cultures, sexual contact is believed to have life-prolonging or invigorating effects. "Although movement therapy offers no encompassing solutions for solving the sexual frustrations of the infirm aged, it does offer opportunities for structured physical contact, mutual caring, and open discussion. Touching and being touched appear to have a rejuvenating effect of the participants which increases their alertness and responsiveness to others. Movement therapy, by humanizing the environment, provides opportunities for geriatric patients to experience their sexuality more freely" (Sandel, 1979, p. 13).

Cardiovascular patients at the onset of recovery need to learn new coping skills for stress management. They face fears and anxieties provoked by what many experience as a betrayal of their bodies. Dance therapy helps the individual to increase body awareness for self-monitoring, self-pacing, and physiological control. At the same time, cardiac rehabilitation program goals encompass physical fitness and a reversal of maladaptive habits that contribute to the original problem.

Chronic pain patients often benefit from learning through dance therapy to be aware of underlying affective states and how they are manifest in pain. Therapists refocus awareness from painful to pleasurable body functions and provide tension-reduction and relaxation techniques to manage the stressors of ongoing pain.

Adolescents experience profound physiological and psychological changes. They attempt to cope with the stresses of the establishment of identity, parental expectations, peer pressures, value conflicts, confused self-image, low self-esteem, unstable body image, emerging sexuality, poor impulse control, and difficulty in interpersonal relations. Dance therapy provides a safe and playful environment in which many areas of conflict can be identified and enacted as well as appropriate adult roles and behavior tried out.

Visually-impaired people are often plagued by the stresses of fantasies and fears stemming from their disabilities (Weisbrod, 1974). Role-playing and the acting out of dreams through movement may be a coping mechanism for many such fears. "For example, Henry, an eleven-year-old, was concerned that because of his poor vision he would not have any friends and would not be invited to any parties. He had created several imaginary friends to the detriment of his real friendships. He was moving very quickly into a make-believe world where everyone liked him. One day in a movement session he acted out going to a party. There he danced and talked with friends but was also rejected by a girl he liked and became sad. Following this event he began an entire series of 'sad' dances. Henry had begun to face his fear and to deal with his sadness.

"Selina was a 10-year-old blind girl who was quite outgoing. She tried to join many of the games and activities of girls on her block. The harder she tried, the more frustrated she became. Her breath became tighter and more shallow. One thing in particular really bothered her. She kept losing the ball or line marker in the games. She eventually began to feel that if she could lose an object so easily, maybe she would get lost and nobody could find her. She began to worry incessantly about being lost and never found. During this time we had been doing a lot of deep breathing. One day she sat very still and did not speak. I asked her what was going on; she shook her head. I left her alone and after a while she began exaggerated grop-ing motions. She called her mother for help. Her breath quickened. I did not answer because I felt she had to work this one out on her own. I trusted what was a kind of basic strength within her. She started crying and crawling across the floor. Finally she started a deep breathing sequence I had taught her and said, 'I am really all by myself. I can find my way on my knees. I am not lost.'

"George, a teen-aged boy, had lost one eye as a child and a year ago had lost the sight of the other eye. Violent and angry parents had caused both losses. He became deeply afraid that someone would come up to him and beat him up. The combined efforts of an under-standing teacher, a blind volunteer worker and myself in movement sessions helped him develop extremely acute hearing so he could hear someone coming and defend himself. In movement sessions we focused on moving aggressively so that he developed his physical and psychic strengths until he could defend himself well.

"Marilyn, who had lost the sight of one eye and had poor vision in the other, feared that birds would come and pluck out her one useful eye. So she played the role of the birds, then of her good eye, and finally of herself. She discovered she could protect herself by shouting and striking out with her arms at the birds. She began to get in touch with her ability to move aggressively.

"Sharon, a 40-year-old totally blind woman institutionalized for additional emotional problems, could not initiate movement. When left alone, she tended to stand still. This is a common ten-dency among congenitally blind people. They lack momentum and initiative to move out on their own. In conjunction with this lack is a tendency to be over-cooperative." Dance therapy helped the woman to get "in touch with her own movement so that she could spontaneously reach out and use space around her in a larger, freer way" (pp. 51–52).

Dance Therapy-Induced Stress

Not only may clients and patients seek or be prescribed dance therapy to resist or reduce stress, but the process of dance therapy may also create stress for the client as mentioned in the introduction. When cultural norms are violated in the dance therapy process, stress is induced rather than alleviated. Touch, for example, has its appropriate use in terms of social status, religious orientation, age, and sex.

There is yet another dimension of induced stress. Therapists themselves seek dance therapy from other therapists in order to deal with the stresses they encounter in their work. Supervision and peer support from people who are aware of the problems are alternative sources of help for the therapist in resisting and reducing the stresses of trying to help clients.

Certain characteristics of the treatment situation with schizophrenic patients stress the therapist (Sandel, 1980). This stress leads the therapist to react with defensive or compensatory responses. These may help the therapist sustain an investment in the patient with a commitment to the treatment process at the same time that the responses may be counterproductive to the patient's treatment. Sandel's work at Yale Psychiatric Institute and her supervision of practicing dance therapists revealed four interrelated issues.

First, the therapist's perceived hopelessness of a treatment situation often leads to the therapist's omnipotent fantasies. This defensive reaction may protect the therapist from feeling despair. However, it may also lead the therapist to perceive improvement in a patient that other clinicians do not see.

Second, the intensity of the therapist's emotional involvement with the patient may make the therapist feel the threat of being overwhelmed. Third, a schizophrenic's lack of responsiveness challenges the therapist's ability to fill up emptiness, to the extent of entertaining the patient. Fourth, the therapist is vulnerable to the effects of the schizophrenics' sensitivity to their unconscious processes. "The therapist's struggle to protect and develop his or her investment in the patient while remaining open to experiencing the hopelessness, anger, and even disorganization stimulated by his or her contact with the patient, emerges in a particular way for the dance therapist. It is affected by both the historical development of dance therapy and the nature of the movement experience" (p. 21).

Sandel recalls a typical experience. She had worked hard during a group therapy session in which all the patients were involved, expressing feelings and creating images. At the end of the session, thinking she was doing a fine job, she asked the group with anticipation how people felt about the session. There was silence. She looked about expectantly, "and one patient said innocently, 'What session?'" (p. 31).

Additionally, therapists who try to help victims of incest tend to feel stress. In her supervisory role, Judith Bunny structures movement exercises to help the therapists meet the pressures of working through the incest victim's family dynamics and emotions.

Commentary

Dance therapy bears resemblances to the therapeutic stress management dance practices found in history and non-Western cultures, past and present. Whereas the former appears to have derived from earlier ritual practices, the various theories of Western dance therapy may illuminate practices of other cultures.

There are a multiplicity of theories, techniques, and clients involved in Western dance therapy. The field is relatively new, but it seems to be increasingly accepted in a host of settings by health practitioners and the general public. This development coincides with the 1960s awareness of the body and research literature on nonverbal communication that has developed, primarily by psychologists, since World War II.

In professional dance, and to a lesser extent amateur dance, the choreographer/dancer chooses to communicate with an audience, be it paying spectators in a theater, a potential sexual partner in a club, or teacher in a studio. By contrast, the patient in dance therapy gives expression to subjective emotion and therapist or other patients may or may not be relevant as receivers of danced messages. The symbol in any kind of dance, however, allows for recall, reenactment, and reexperience of events for purposes of resisting, reducing, transforming, and escaping stress.

Chapter 12
Conclusion: Stress and Dance Patterns

Why Dance?

The configuration of human behavior that is called dance has its roots in phylogeny (development of the living species) and ontogeny (development of the individual). Humans have predispositions to dance that are shaped by social experience. The physical, affective, and cognitive properties of dance described in the introduction suggest its potential in promoting health. There is data on dance and stress reported by observers, although little is scientifically tested, and the relation of dance and stress or other physical fitness training evidence is based on association rather than demonstrated causality (Morgan, 1984). Yet, the persistence of dance since the times of early humanity attests to its efficacy in helping people to resist, reduce, and escape stress.

There is no question that there are alternative ways of dealing with stress. Some are passive, such as meditation, yoga, repetitive prayer, biofeedback, or progressive muscle relaxation that break the train of everyday thought and decrease the activity of the sympathetic nervous system. Other ways of managing stress are active. Exercise has been shown to have chronic or long-term effects in developing physical fitness, providing outlets for pent-up tension, reducing anxiety, developing higher tolerance levels for stress, and so on. Exercise utilizes the potentially harmful biochemical elements of energy released into the body when it mobilizes against stress in the fight or flight response and the individual is in a situation where this energy must be contained. Physical fitness abets a positive state of mental health which resists disease. As with many health problems, it is less costly in time, money, and effort to prevent disabling effects of stress than to arrest or cure them.

If one selects an active mode, why choose dance over other forms of physical exercise as part of one's repertoire of stress management techniques? Exercise such as biking or running can cause imbalance in the muscles and joints of the body (Alter, 1983). These activities which maintain cardiovascular fitness mainly contract muscles. Selected forms of dancing provide stretching as well.

The material presented in this book attests to the fact that dance is more than physical exercise for fitness. Dance is a result of physical as well as affective and mental processes. A kinetic discourse directed by the same cognitive processes that operate in verbal language, dance is commonly communication, the symbolic visualizations embodied in the dancer who engages in self-mastery. Sometimes dance action also allows mastery over others, holding the self and/or the world up to critical scrutiny and shaping one or the other in a desired manner. Dance permits emotional and intellectual exploration in addition to aesthetic involvement and movement satisfaction.

A medium for the secular mediation of stress, dance is also a mode of spirituality (personal experience toward connection with the numinous) or religiosity (experience of organized religion) that helps order one's life. Moreover, we know that health care and curing are inseparable from the total history of communal organization and of economy. Disease may not be an individual affliction but a malady that emerges from social conditions. The dance may be a vehicle for manifestation of divinity and a bringing together of family and community, in reality or fantasy. Additionally, dance is usually accompanied by music which offers people gratification and functions in ways similar to dance.

Dance is not a single entity, but a variety of genres and subtypes that function in manifold ways for different kinds of participants. One can be an amateur, a professional dancer or a client in a dance therapy situation. Furthermore, a cross-cultural perspective reveals an infinite variety of corporeal techniques embedded in cultural and social contexts. Sometimes dance triggers stress that enables an individual to deal with greater stressors; at other times dance calms and buoys a stressed individual. Some people go into trance while dancing; others dance to get out of trance as when a deity incarnates itself within a particular person, who becomes its vessel. No single explanation fits for dance-stress relationships.

In spite of its benefits, dance may not be appropriate for everyone. Some individuals have strong negative attitudes toward dance because of religious training or social upbringing, traumatic experience in the activity, or associations of dance with specific gender roles and behavior. Physical limitations may also counterindicate dancing. Using dance as an accommodation to stress through the discharge of tension or withdrawal or escape from stress through altered states of consciousness could preclude or retard the resolution of a problem.

Guidelines for Preventing, Reducing, or Escaping Stress through Dance

For success in avoiding or reducing stress by dancing, one must decide that dancing is important. This book supports such a decision. However, which dance genre provides the greatest benefit is unclear. Much depends upon the individual and his or her own mind, body, and experience in the context of daily activity, dance instruction, and specific society and culture. Professional dancers need supplementary dance exercise outside the studio rehearsal hall, and theater to enhance fitness and endurance. Endurance is important after several hours of dance technique classes followed by rehearsal and performance, because many injuries result from fatigue. Lowered heart rate improves the dancer's ability to handle stress.

Physical Guidelines. Much of what doctors prescribe for exercise in health and disease generally is applicable to dancing. Paradoxically, the pursuit of better health through exercise too often results in unnecessary injury and impaired health. Physical injury is always a possibility. However, there are ways to make dancing less risky. These considerations (taken from Alter, 1983, 1986; Pollock, Wilmore, and Fox, 1984; and Shell, 1986) directly influence the success or failure of dance in a stress management program.

A person's *physical fitness* and *age* are certainly important in selecting the level for a dance/stress program and the rate of progression. It is critical to take into account one's medical history and risk associated with having coronary artery disease. A medical examination may be necessary before a sedentary person embarks upon a dance program. Dancing for older adults requires special care because of the dire medical consequences of physical stress. Stress testing for someone who does not usually dance is recommended. Treadmill, bicycle, and step tests are used for this purpose (Smith and Serfass, 1981). Heart patients need to be aware that opium-like, pain-killing brain chemicals, beta endorphins, associated with the "runners' high" or exhilaration, could be hiding symptoms of dangerous heart damage, according to David Sheps's research (reported at the 1986 American Heart Association). It is preferable that heart patients feel the stress on their hearts so that they can reduce their activity appropriately.

For the nonprofessional, beginning a dance program gradually and using *moderation* are keys to preventing physical stress. Dancing regularly, from three to five days per week with conditioning every other day, is recommended for fitness. A regimen of exercise coupled with rest time between workouts for the musculoskeletal system to adapt is most likely to build endurance and prevent injury. This pattern provides immediate physical reinforcement as well as long-term benefit.

The *climatic environment* in which people dance influences their ability to perform successfully. High temperature, humidity, and radiation from the sun combined with low air movement and dancer acclimatization put stress on the dancer if the movement is intense and of long duration. Dehydration, or body water loss from exercising in the heat, if not attended to with ingestion of water or a diluted electrolyte solution for quick rehydration, can result in heat exhaustion or stroke. Since dancing itself provides considerable body heat and additional clothing can be worn, exercise in the cold presents fewer problems. The body does take a longer time to warm up, however. In certain areas of the United States air pollution, especially high concentrations of carbon monoxide and ozone, can have a negative effect on dancing. When pollution reaches the "air alert" stage, no exercise is recommended. People unaccustomed to high altitudes find their bodies have difficulty in delivering oxygen to working muscles and thus movement capacity diminishes. Floor surfaces should have resilience to avoid leg and back injuries.

Clothing and *shoes* are important. Overdress or underdressing or wearing the wrong size or type of shoe can cause serious problems of climatic stress, disability or injury. Doctors say, "under no circumstances should one exercise while wearing rubberized or plastic clothing. . . . The increased sweat loss does not result in a permanent loss of body weight. . . . The . . . clothing does not allow the body sweat to evaporate. Since sweating is the principal manner in which the body regulates its temperature during exercise, lack of sweating or reduced evaporation of sweat can lead to a dramatic increase in body temperature, excessive dehydration and salt loss, and possible heat stroke or heat exhaustion" (Pollock et al., 1984, p. 375).

Some dancing, such as modern and Afro-Caribbean, calls for barefoot action. Until the bottoms of the *feet* toughen and develop protective callouses, beginners may develop blisters. A toe box in any shoe with insufficient clearance between the toes and the underside of the toe box may cause black toenails as a result of blood blisters that form under the toenail. Tap, jazz, ballet, and toe shoes require proper fitting that is usually found in specialized dance supply stores. For example, leather jazz shoes are at first supposed to feel very tight since the leather stretches as one dances. For aerobics dancing a shoe with good shock-absorbing qualities and lateral support is desirable. Of course, a resilient floor (wood or special composition) rather than concrete is important in preventing foot and leg injury.

A dance session, class, or activity should begin with a *warm-up*, preferably until the body perspires, and end with a cool-down to prevent bodily injury such as muscle pulls, strains, sprains, and lower back discomfort, as well as reducing the extent of muscle soreness. Stretching exercises develop and maintain flexibility in addition to preparing the muscles, joints, and ligaments for dancing. Moreover, sudden vigorous exercise places a potentially lethal strain on the heart.

After vigorous dancing, the *cool-down* period with light movement and stretching exercises that involve the legs and lower back keeps the primary muscle groups which were involved in the endurance exercise continuously active and helps to prevent extreme muscle soreness. Exercises that involve the legs and are typically performed in an upright position will cause blood to pool in the lower half of the body if the individual does not perform light activity, such as walking or similar locomotion, during the recovery period. This activity allows the leg muscles to assist the return of the pooled blood to the heart, which, in turn, provides an adequate blood flow to the brain. Abrupt stopping of dancing and inadequate blood flow to the brain could cause dizziness and even passing out. Following a dancing workout a warm, rather than a hot, shower is recommended. The latter can create the cardiovascular complications of peripheral dilation of blood pooling.

Dancers need to be aware of *signals* from their *bodies* to avoid physical stress, injury, and even death. They should have realistic expectations about what they can do within a given period of time, the constraints of body build, and prior experience. Suffering previous injuries alerts one to potential weaknesses and recurrences. Living past the age of 35 means that there is a chance of bodily wear and tear in parts of the body predisposing them to a breakdown with overexertion. If a person has a vulnerable area, massage or heat with warm water will loosen the muscles and increase the blood supply.

Warning signs and symptoms could occur either during or immediately after exercise; what is applicable to jogging is applicable to dancing (Sachs and Buffone, 1984). Abnormal heart activity (irregular pulse, either a sudden burst of rapid heartbeats or a slow pulse falling rapidly), a pain or pressure in the chest, arm or throat, sudden lack of coordination, confusion, cold sweating, pallor, a purplish discoloration of the skin due to deficient oxygenation of the blood, and fainting indicate one should stop dancing and see a physician before resuming exercise. Dancing should be avoided when fever is present since viral infections can possibly infect the heart muscle.

Some signs that occur during or after exercise suggest the dancer take corrective measures to prevent injury. If such problems do not disappear with remedial action, then a physician consultation is appropriate. For a rapid pulse rate that persists throughout five to ten minutes of recovery or longer, the dancer should reduce the intensity of dancing and progress to higher levels at a slower rate. Nausea or vomiting after dancing may require a reduced intensity of the endurance exercise and prolonged cool-down period as well as avoidance of eating for at least two hours prior to dancing. Extreme breathlessness lasting more than ten minutes after ceasing to dance and prolonged fatigue up to 24 hours after exercise may respond to reducing the intensity of dancing.

Blisters from dancing with tender feet or new shoes, should be punctured at the edge with a sterile needle to drain the fluid and then covered with a topical antiseptic and bandage.

Muscle *soreness* usually accompanies a change in exercise habits. Discomfort may occur during the latter stages of dancing, during immediate recovery, and between 12 and 48 hours after strenuous exercise. The soreness can be reduced by the warm-up/cool down approach suggested above as well as massage and warm baths. Muscle cramp, involuntary muscle contractions possibly the result of a salt and potassium imbalance in the muscle, can be relieved by stretching and massaging.

For bone *bruises* on the bottoms of the feet caused by jumping or leaping, ice and padding on the area provide some relief. Knee pain and shin splits (a sharp pain on the front of the tibia, probably due to factors such as a lowered arch, hairline or stress fracture of the bone, and tearing of the muscle where it attaches to bone) usually respond to rest and limited dancing with the knee or leg wrapped. Dancers may injure the achilles tendon or ankle. Putting ice on the injured area immediately prevents major swelling and facilitates recovery through rest or reduced activity.

Some individuals have used dancing to highly *titrate*, or tune, their bodies and minds to bring about a given effect, usually of feeling good, energetic, and productive. This dance program works for them most of the time. However, when an accident occurs that prevents the customary dancing, the individual may experience more stress than otherwise (titrating observations, orthopedic surgeon, Walter Abendschein, April 7, 1986).

In selecting a dance/therapy program, it is important to have a *trained instructor/therapist* who understands kinesiology and is sensitive to individual needs. Sometimes teachers teach what they were taught or what works for their own bodies even though it contradicts contemporary knowledge about healthy practice.

Professional dancers need to be aware of the danger of excessive *thinness* and vigorous exercise. This combination, which disrupts the menstrual cycle and lowers estrogen levels, can endanger fertility, decrease the body's ability to utilize calcium, interfere with bone mineral content, and increase the risk of bone injury.

The *level of dance activity* a person undertakes has implications for stress. Selection of dance activities that are too simple may lead to boredom. Activities that are demanding tend to be regarded as stimulating and energizing. However, if they are too demanding they may tax a person's coping ability and elicit high levels of anxiety and reduced effort, fatigue, exhaustion, and burn-out. If you do not like one class or teacher (personality, selection of music, or style of instruction), try another. Experiment with different forms of dance and varying levels of difficulty.

Cognitive Guidelines. Dancers can draw upon a variety of techniques to cope with performance anxiety and fear and to improve performance which, in turn, often decreases "stage fright." *Biofeedback* help individuals assess their own internal stress responses through, for example, muscle tension, skin temperature, sweat activity, elevated heart rate, and dry mouth. *Meditation* techniques such as transcendental meditation (TM), yoga, and Zen may be used to induce relaxation before a performance and to promote improved concentration for body control. *Positive thinking* and *autogenics* involve verbalizing a desired outcome so that performance anxiety is allayed.

Imagery (formerly known as mental practice) refers to visualizing oneself performing a skill, rehearsing it in one's mind prior to its actual execution (Magill, 1985, pp. 389–92); Overby, 1986). There is either a mental image in our brain or the graphic and detailed nature of language makes it seem so. Imaging a dance action initiates electrical impulses along certain neurological pathways to the musculature that is involved in the movement and thus activates the movement and inhibits impulses to other muscles. Internal imagery is the imagination of the kinesthetic experience of the correct performance of a movement. External imagery is the visualization of oneself performing the movement.

Visual-motor behavior rehearsal (VMBR) combines relaxation and imagery. Going through stressful experiences mentally should make it easier to deal with the stress of actual performance.

Body therapies, drawing upon visualizing accurate images of intended movements, augment injury-prevention activities as well as rehabilitation between the end of medical treatment and the return to skilled performance (Meyers, 1986a, 1986b). Alexander technique, Feldenkrais awareness through movement, Laban/Bartenieff movement analysis and fundamentals, Rolfing integration of human structure, Silver's sensory awareness, Todd/Sweigard ideokinetic facilitation, Jacobson's progressive relaxation, Trager Psychophysical Integration, Ashton patterning, Bioenergetics, and Bonnie Cohen's Mind/Body Centering are some of the therapy principles and interventions. They attempt to draw awareness to maladaptive automatic motor habits in order to discover new and more effective patterns of, for example, body alignment, breathing patterns, and mechanical balance.

Guidelines for Analyzing Meaning in Movement

In order to understand meaning in movement for dance therapy (in diagnosing problems, measuring change, and interpreting client insights mediated through dance) and for observers of dance in exotic societies or their own theaters, a semantic grid is a useful tool. I developed this tool in trying to discover meaning in Nigeria's

Ubakala dance and analyze it in cross-cultural perspective (Hanna, 1979b, 1987d).

Although there are several notation systems that describe movement as motion, none refers to what the movements signify or offers direction in identifying such meaning, what a thing or an idea stands for. Meaning is communication in contexts with shared semantics among dancers and observers. Meaning also may be found in dance when the dancer has no intention to communicate. Meaning may lie in the rules dictating how signs may be combined, that is, the grammar; a different way of saying something (how) may be saying a different thing (what).

To probe for meaning, the grid can be imposed on the whole dance and used to zoom in on smaller units as one turns a telescope lens in order to bring images into focus. Placing each unit of dance within each cell of the grid matrix permits the confrontation of the possibility (existence/nonexistence) of forms of encoding meaning and the transformation of these over time. Let us turn to the grid (see Figure 1, and read vertically). Six *devices* that have been found in a global survey of dance are presented for conveying meaning. Each device may be conventional (customary shared legacy) or autographic (idiosyncratic or creative expression of a thing, event, or condition).

(1) A *concretization* produces the outward aspect of a thing, event, or condition; for example, mimetically portraying a battle. It is an imitation. (2) An *icon* represents most properties of a thing, event, or condition, and is responded to as if it were what it represents. An illustration is dancing the role of a deity who is revered or otherwise treated as the deity. The Haitians believe Ghede appears when a dancer is possessed by him, and they treat the dancer in this state with genuine awe. (3) A *stylization* encompasses somewhat arbitrary gestures or movements that are the result of convention. In ballet pointing to the heart is a sign of love. (4) A *metonym* is a motional conceptualization of one thing for that of another of which it is an attribute or extension, or with which it is associated or contiguous in the same frame of experience. A war dance as part of a battle is a case in point. (5) A *metaphor* expresses

Figure 1 Semantic Grid

DEVICES	SPHERES				Intermesh with	Vehicle for		
	Event	Whole Body	Discursive Performance	Specific Performance	Movement	Other Medium	Other Medium	Presence
Concretization c	– –	– –	– –	– –	– –	– –	– –	– –
a								
Icon c	– –	– –	– –	– –	– –	– –	– –	– –
a								
Stylization c	– –	– –	– –	– –	– –	– –	– –	– –
a								
Metonym c	– –	– –	– –	– –	– –	– –	– –	– –
a								
Metaphor c	– –	– –	– –	– –	– –	– –	– –	– –
a								
Actualization c	– –	– –	– –	– –	– –	– –	– –	– –
a								

c = Conventional
a = Autographical

one thought, experience, or phenomenon in place of another which resembles the former to suggest an analogy between the two. Dancing the role of a leopard to denote the power of death is an example. (6) An *actualization* is an individual dancing one or several of his usual statuses and roles such as Louis XIV dancing the role of king and being so treated.

Meaning usually depends on context. The devices for encapsulating meaning seem to operate within one or more of eight spheres (read the grid horizontally): (1) the sociocultural *event* and/or situation; (2) the total human *body* in action; (3) the whole pattern of the *performance*; (4) the *discursive* aspect of the performance (the *sequence* of unfolding movement configurations); (5) specific *movement*; (6) the *intermesh* of movement with other communication media (for example, dance meaning being inseparable from song, music, costume, accoutrement and/or speech); (7) dance movement as a *vehicle* for another medium (for example, dance providing background for a performer's poetry recitation); and (8) *presence* (the emotional turn-on through projected sensuality or charisma).

Singly or in combination the devices and spheres allow for consideration of all message material in terms of possible relations to context. The devices are signs that may function as signals when they are directly related to the action they signify, such as a war dance to herald a battle. Valid semantic analyses largely depend on dance data collection procedures. The use of multiple approaches helps to overcome the problems of reliance on a single one. Relevant considerations are (1)how movers use movement and relate to each other in the process, (2) what the movers and observers say about the movement, and (3) how movement symbols relate to other symbols used by the individual and by his or her society. It is important to consider the range of semantic complexity such as tacit knowledge, hierarchical levels of meaning, use of opposites and inversions, ambiguity, synonyms, changing meaning of a device at different phases in performance, and operation of metaphoric equations in two directions at once. Illustratively, if one is dancing Dylan Thomas's "our eunuch dreams," one needs to know not only that a eunuch is a man who has been castrated, but also that castration destroys sexual potency, and that sexual potency is to be taken as a symbol of efficacy in general. Saying the lion is king of the beasts says something about lions and also something about kings.

Commentary

This book has explored patterns of dance and stress, how dance may be a means through which people resist, reduce, induce, and escape stress. The work has taken a broad view of past and present and near and far cultures.

Dance has kaleidoscopic variety and complexity. Yet, in contemporary secular and Western therapeutic dance, as in other ritual modalities, in order to manage stress people meet demons; shake off death, sin, and evil; come to terms with life crises; mediate paradoxes; resolve conflict; revitalize the past to recreate the present; enhance their self-concept and body image; attract attention; assert themselves; confront the strong; and persuade others to change their ways. Every society attempts to define stress and to explain its causes and proper responses. When social conflict causes stress, the "therapy" tends to be group-related with an interactional script. Danced healing rituals (in African village compounds, temple courtyards, dance therapy studios, public theaters, and other social settings) reinvoke old traumas for exorcism and the transformation of fear, convince people that evil is gone or possible to dissipate, and reaffirm communal solidarity. Disclosure through personal introspection, masked demon dancing, or other supernatural revelation is to expose to therapeutic action.

In the interweave of mind and body, dance is a mode that allows people to work through difficulties, anticipate the future, recollect the past, and confront the present. Participants in dance, both dancers and viewers, may experience catharsis and develop a sense of mastery or self-discovery. Moreover, movers may achieve physical fitness that ameliorates fatigue, aging, premenstrual discomfort, and disease. Whether tarantism or contemporary amateur or professional theater art, the dance medium gives scope for self-expression and opportunity for approbation. Dance often has an affective contagion, whether manifest in Zulu mobilization for war or American marathon defense against depression.

In sum, dance may be pleasurable in and of itself; it may, however, also move individuals to personal and social action beyond the dance setting. Prophylactic against the negative affects of stress and remediative in transforming distress, dance has unique potential.

Little research has been conducted in the kinds of relationships between dance and stress. It is my hope that this book will stimulate further exploration in order to generate knowledge that will help people better cope with stress in modern society and attain the exquisite balance of being.

References

Aaron, S. (1986). *Stage fright: Its role in acting*. Chicago: University of Chicago Press.

Abrams, G. L. (1985–86). "Report on the First International Conference on Mind, Body and the Performing Arts: Stress processes in the psychology and physiology of music, dance and drama, New York University, July 15–19, 1985." *Dance Research Journal*, 17 (2) & 18 (1).

Adams, C. (1986). "Collaboration: An artist's view." *Update Dance/USA*, 4 (1): 8.

Akstein, D. (1973). "Terpsichoreotrancetherapy: A new hypopsychotherapeutic method." *International Journal of Clinical and Experimental Hypnosis*, 21 (3): 131–143.

Alliance for the Arts (1985). *Spaces for the arts: A study of the real estate needs of non-profit arts organizations in New York City*. New York: Alliance for the Arts.

Alter, J. (1983). *Surviving exercise*. Boston: Houghton Mifflin.

Alter, J. (1986). *Stretch and strengthen*. Boston: Houghton Mifflin.

Amoss, P. (1978). *Coast Salish Spirit Dancing: The survival of an ancestral religion*. Seattle: University of Washington Press.

Anderson, D. (1985). "Eating disorders." *Update Dance/USA*, 3 (7): 9–11.

Anderson, J. (1986). "Dance: D. J. McDonald explores growing old." *New York Times*, February 26, p. C1.

Andrews, E. A. (1940). *The gift to be simple: Songs, dances and rituals of the American Shakers*. New York: Dover.

Angioli, M. D. (1982). *Body image perception and locus of control in semi-nude and nude female dancers*. Doctoral dissertation, United States International University. Ann Arbor: University Microfilms.

Backman, E. L. (1952). *Religious dances in the Christian church and in popular medicine*. Trans. E. Classen. London: George Allen & Unwin Ltd.

Behavioral Medicine (1979). "Stressful living country-style." 6 (2): 36–39.

Bentley, T. (1982). *Winter season: A dancer's journal*. New York: Random House.

Bentley, T. (1986). "Reaching for perfection—the life and death of a dancer." *New York Times*, April 17, pp. H1, 25.

Berger, B. G. (1984). "Running away from anxiety and depression: A female as well as male race." In M. L. Sachs and G. W. Buffone (eds.), *Running as therapy: An integrated approach* (pp. 138–171). Lincoln: University of Nebraska Press.

Bernstein, P. (1979). *Eight theoretical approaches in dance-movement therapy*. Dubuque, Iowa: Kendall Hunt.

Blum, L. H. (1966–67). "The discotheque and the phenomenon of alone-togetherness." *Adolescence*, 1 (4): 351–366.

Braiker, H. (1986). "The Type E woman: How to overcome the stress of being everything to everybody." Nashville, Tenn.: Dodd Mead.

Brierly, H. (1979). *Transvestism*. Oxford: Pergamon Press.

Brody, J. E. (1986a). "Personal health." *New York Times*, April 16, p. C10.

———. (1986b). "Moderate exercise late in life is found to reverse many of the effects of aging." *New York Times*, June 10, p. C1, 3.

Bullough, V. L. (1976). *Sexual variance in society and history*. Chicago: University of Chicago Press.

Bychowski, G. (1951). "From catharsis to work of art: The making of an artist." In G. B. Wilbur and W. Muensterberger (eds.), *Psychoanalysis and culture: Essays in honor of Geza Roheim* (pp. 390–409). New York: International Universities Press.

Calabria, F. M. (1976). "The dance marathon craze." *Journal of Popular Culture*, 10, (1):54–69.

Cannon, W. B. (1929). *Bodily changes in pain, hunger, fear and rage* (2nd ed.). New York: D. Appleton.

Cannon, W. B. (1932). *The wisdom of the body*. New York: W. W. Norton.

Chilivumbo, A. (1969). "Some traditional Malawi dances: A preliminary account." Mimeographed.

Chryst, G. (1986). Interview by Effie Mihopoulos. *Salome*, 44/45/46, pp. 44–48.

Cooper, K. H. (1970). *The new aerobics.* New York: Bantam.

Crapanzano, V. (1973). *The Hamadsha: A study in Moroccan ethnopsychiatry.* Berkeley: University of California Press.

Csikszentmihalyi, M. (1975). *Beyond boredom and anxiety: The experience in work and games.* San Francisco: Jossey Bass.

Delaney, W. (1982). "Dance therapy in evaluation and treatment." In H. S. Moffic and G. L. Adams (eds.), *A clinician's manual on mental health care* (pp. 154–160). Menlo Park, Calif.: Addison-Wesley.

de Martino, E. (1966). *La terre du remords.* Trans. by C. Poncet. Paris: Gallimard.

de Mille, A. (1960). *To a young dancer: A handbook for dance students, parents, and teachers.* Boston: Little, Brown & Co.

Dorward, D. C., ed. (1982). *The Igbo Women's War of 1929: Documents relating to the Aba Riots in Eastern Nigeria.* New York: Microform, Ltd., Clearwater Publications.

Dow, J. (1986). "Universal aspects of symbolic healing: A theoretical synthesis." *Current Anthropology,* 88 (1):56–69.

Dunning, J. (1986). "Dance: Eleo Pomare Troupe on Mandela theme." *New York Times,* February 24, p. C13.

———. (1987). "Eviction for Erick Hawkins." *New York Times,* May 30, p. 13.

Dutton, D. (1977). "Art, behavior, and the anthropologists." *Current Anthropology,* 18, 387–407.

English, H. B. & English, A. C. (1958). *A comprehensive dictionary of psychological and psychoanalytic terms.* New York: McKay.

Farrer, C. R. (1976). "Play and inter-ethnic communication." In D. Lancy and B. A. Tindal (eds.), *The anthropological study of play* (pp. 86–92). Cornwall, N.Y.: Leisure Press.

Fenichel, O. (1972). *The psychoanalytic theory of neurosis.* New York: W. W. Norton.

Fergusson, E. (1931). *Dancing gods: Indian ceremonials of New Mexico and Arizona.* Albuquerque: University of New Mexico Press.

Fernandez, J. (1982). *Bwiti: An ethnography of the religious imagination in Africa.* Princeton: Princeton University Press.

Forman, J. S. (1983). *The effects of an aerobic dance program for women teachers on symptoms of burnout.* Unpublished doctoral dissertation, University of Cincinnati.

Forsyth, S., & Kolenda, P. M. (1966). "Competition, cooperation, and group cohesion in the ballet company." *Psychiatry,* 29 (2): 123–145.

Foulks, E. F., Wintrob, R. M., Westermeyer, J., & Favazza, A. R. (eds.). (1977). *Current perspectives in cultural psychiatry.* New York: Spectrum.

Frank, J. E. (1973). *Persuasion and healing: A comparative study of psychotherapy* (rev. ed.). Baltimore: Johns Hopkins University Press.

Freud, S. (1955). *Beyond the pleasure principle.* London: Hogarth Press.

Gailey, H. A. (1970). *The road to Aba: A study of British administrative policy in Eastern Nigeria.* New York: New York University Press.

Gardner, H. (1983). *Frames of mind: A theory of multiple intelligences.* New York: Basic Books.

Gazzaniga, M. (1985). "The social brain." *Psychology Today,* 19 (1): 29–30, 32–34, 36–37.

Glaser, R. (1986). *Modulation of the immune response during stress.* Paper presented at the conference on Mechanisms of Physical and Emotional Stress, National Institutes of Health, Bethesda, Md.

Gordon, S. (1983). *Off balance: The real world of ballete.* New York: Pantheon.

Griaule, M. (1965). *Conversations with Ogotemmeli: An introduction to Dogon religious ideas.* London: Oxford University Press.

Gruen, J. (1986). "Bruhn on Bruhn." *Dancemagazine,* 56 (6): 33.

Guenther, M. G. (1975). "The trance dancer as an agent of social change among the farm Bushmen of the Ghanzi district." *Botswana Notes and Records,* 7: 161–166.

Hager, B. (1978). *The dancer's world: Problems of today and tomorrow.* Report of the First International Choreographers' Conference. np: UNESCO Cultural Development Documentary Dossier 20.

Halpern, R. H. (1981). *Female occupational exhibitionism: An exploratory study of topless and bottomless dancers.* Doctoral dissertation, United States International University. Ann Arbor: University Microfilms.

Hanna, J. L. (1976). *The anthropology of dance ritual: Nigeria's Ubakala nkwa di iche iche.* Doctoral dissertation, Columbia University. Ann Arbor: University Microfilms.

————. (1979a). "Movements toward understanding humans through the anthropological study of dance." *Current Anthropology,* 20 (2): 313–339.

————. (1979b). "Toward semantic analysis of movement behavior: Concepts and problems." *Semiotica,* 25 (1–2): 77–110.

————. (1982). "Public policy and the children's world: Implications of ethnographic research for desegregated schooling." In G. D. Spindler (ed.), *Doing the ethnography of schooling: Educational anthropology in action* (pp. 316–355). New York: Holt, Rinehart and Winston.

_____. (1983). *The performer-audience connection: Emotion to metaphor in dance and society.* Austin: University of Texas Press.

_____. (1984). "Towards discovering the universals of dance." *World of Music,* 26 (2): 88–103.

_____. (1985). "The impact of the critic: Comments from the critics and the criticized." In J. Robinson (ed.), *Social science and the arts, 1984* (pp. 141–162). Lanham, Md.: University Press of America.

_____. (1986a). "Movement in African performance." In B. Fleshman (ed.), *Theatrical movement: A bibliographical anthology* (pp. 561–585). Metuchen, N.J.: Scarecrow Press.

_____. (1986b). "Interethnic communication in children's own dance, play, and protest." In Young Y. Kim (ed.), *Interethnic Communication* (Vol. 10, International and Intercultural Communication Annual, pp. 176–198). Newbury Park, Calif.: Sage Publications.

_____. (1987a). "Dance: Dance and religion." In M. Eliade (ed.),*The encyclopedia of religion* (Vol. 4, pp. 203–212). New York: Macmillan Co.

_____. (1987b). "Gender 'language' onstage; Moves, new moves and countermoves." *Journal of the Washington Academy of Sciences,* 77 (1): 18–26.

_____. (1987c). "Patterns of dominance: Male, female, and homosexuality in dance." *The Drama Review,* 113, 31 (1): 24–47.

_____. (1987d). *To dance is human: A theory of nonverbal communication.* Chicago: University of Chicago Press (orig. 1979. Austin: University of Texas Press).

_____. (1988a). "The representation and reality of divinity in dance." *Journal of the American Academy of Religion,* Vol. 56: (2).

_____. (1988b). *Disruptive school behavior: Class, race, and culture.* New York: Holmes & Meier.

_____. (1988c). *Dance, sex, and gender: Signs of identity, dominance, defiance, and desire.* Chicago: University of Chicago Press.

Hanna, J. L. & Hanna, W. J. (1968). "Nkwa di iche iche: Dance-plays of Ubakala." *Presence Africaine,* 65: 13–38.

Hansen, C. (1967). "Jenny's toes: Negro shaking dances in America." *American Quarterly,* 19, 554–63.

Harre, R. & Lamb, R. (1983). *Encyclopedic dictionary of psychology.* Cambridge, Mass.: MIT Press.

Hendin, J. & Csikszentmihalyi, M. (1975). "Measuring the flow experience in rock dancing." In M. Csikszentmihalyi, M., *Beyond boredom and anxiety* (pp. 102–122). San Francisco: Jossey Bass.

Hoerburger, F. (1965). "Folk dance survey." *Journal of the International Folk Music Council,* 17 (part 1): 7–8.

Holcomb, J. M. (1977). *The effects of dancing and relaxation sessions on stress levels of senior citizens.* Unpublished doctoral dissertation, United States International University.

Horosko, M. (1986). "Health: doctors for dancers." *Dancemagazine,* 55 (5): 106.

Horton, R. (1960). *The gods as guests: An aspect of Kalabari religious life.* Lagos: Nigeria Magazine Special Publication.

Howard, J. H. (1983). "Pan-Indianism in native American music and dance." *Ethnomusicology,* 27 (1): 71–82.

Ilogu, E. (1965). "Christianity and Ibo traditional religion." *International Revue of Missions,* 54 (215): 335–342.

Jackson, G. (1978). *Dance as dance: Selected reviews and essays.* Ontario, Canada: Catalyst.

Jacob, E. (1981). *Dancing: A guide for the dancer you can be.* Reading, Mass.: Addison-Wesley.

Jones, B., & Hawes, B. L. (1972). *Step it down: Games, plays and stories from the Afro-American heritage.* New York: Harper & Row.

Kapferer, B. A. (1983). *A celebration of demons: Exorcism and the aesthetics of healing in Sri Lanka.* Bloomington: Indiana University Press.

Katch, F. I., & McArdle, W. D. (1977). *Nutrition, weight control, and exercise.* Boston: Houghton Mifflin.

Kealiinohomoku, J. (1969–70). "An anthropologist looks at ballet as a form of ethnic dance." *Impulse: Extensions of dance,* pp. 24–33.

Keleman, S. (1975). *Living your dying.* New York: Random House.

Kendall, L. (1985). *Shamans, housewives, and other restless spirits: Women in Korean ritual life.* Honolulu: University of Hawaii Press.

Kern, L. (1981). *An ordered love: Sex roles and sexuality in Victorian utopias: the Shakers, the Mormons, and the Oneida Community.* Chapel Hill: University of North Carolina Press.

Kiecolt-Glaser, J. (1986). *Psycho-social influence on the immune response.* Paper presented at the conference on Mechanisms of Physical and Emotional Stress, National Institutes of Health, Bethesda, Md.

Kirkland, G. (1986). *Dancing on my grave.* New York: Doubleday.

Kisselgoff, A. (1982). "Forsythe's 'Say Bye-bye' startles and excites." *New York Times,* August 1, p. H8.

Kriegsman, A. M. (1987). "The Dance Theatre of Harlem. Steps ahead at the Kennedy Center Opera House, Garth Fagan's 'Footprints'." *Washington Post,* February 15, pp. F1, 10–11.

Lamb, D. R. (1978). *Physiology of exercise.* New York: Macmillan.

Lambo, T. A. (1965). "The place of the arts in the emotional life of the African." *AMSAC Newsletter,* 7 (4): 1–6.

Lee, R. B. (1967). "Trance cure of the !Kung bushman." *Natural History,* 76 (a): 31–37.

Lerman, L. (1984). *Teaching dance to senior adults.* Springfield, Ill.: Charles C. Thomas.

Levanthal, M. B. (ed., Compiled by Council of Graduate Dance/ Movement Therapy Educators). (1983). *Graduate research and studies in dance/movement therapy 1972–82.* Philadelphia: Hahnemann University Press.

Levine, L. W. (1977). *Culture and black consciousness: Afro-American folk thought from slavery to freedom.* New York: Oxford University Press.

Lopata, H. Z., & Noel, J. (1972). "The dance studio—style without sex." In G. P. Stone (ed.), *Games, sport and power* (pp. 184–201). New Brunswick: Transaction Books.

McElroy, A., & Townsend, P. K. (1979). *Medical anthropology in ecological perspective.* North Scituate, Mass.: Duxbury Press.

McIntyre, M. (1986). "Resisting the recognizable." *Washington Post,* June 2, p. B7.

McKean, P. F. (1979). "From purity to pollution: The Balinese Ketjak (monkey dance) as symbolic form in transition." In A. L. Becker and A. A. Yenogyan (eds.), *The imagination of reality* (pp. 293–302). Norwood, N.J.: Ablex.

McNees, P. (1987). "Diversions: Folk dancing's leaps and bounds: Every night, there's action." *Washington Post,* February 6, p. C5.

Madsen, W. (1973). *Mexican-Americans of South Texas* (2nd ed.). New York: Holt, Rinehart and Winston.

Magill, R. A. (1985). *Motor learning concepts and applications.* Dubuque, Iowa: Wm. C. Brown.

Manning, P. K., and Fabrega, H. Jr. (1973). "The experience of self and body: health and illness in the Chiapas highlands." In *Phenomenological sociology: Issues and applications* (pp. 251–301). New York: Wiley.

Marshall, L. (1962). "!Kung Bushman religious beliefs." *Africa,* 32: 221–252.

Martin, C. (ed.). (1986). "Life on the floor: Art, sport, and scam: Dance marathons of the twenties and thirties." *New Observations,* #39.

Mason, K. C. (ed.). (1974). *Therapy: Focus on Dance VII.* Washington, D.C.: American Association for Health, Physical Education and Recreation.

Mazo, J. H. (1974). *Dance is a contact sport*. New York: Dutton.

Medical Problems of Performing Artists. (1986). "Coping with stress: Roundtable discussion." 1 (1): 12–16.

Meek, C. K. (1931). *Tribal studies in northern Nigeria*. London: Kegan Paul, Trench, Trubner.

Meek, C. K. (1937). *Law and authority in a Nigerian tribe*. London: Oxford University Press.

Merton, R. K. (1957). *Social theory and social structure*. Glencoe, Ill.: Free Press.

Meyers, M. (1986a). "Perceptual awareness in integrative movement behavior: The role of integrative movement systems (body therapies) in motor performance and expressivity." In C. G. Shell (ed.), *The dancer as athlete* (pp. 163–186). Champaign, Ill.: Human Kinetics Publishers.

Meyers, M., Pierpont, M., & Schnitt, D. (1986b). "Body systems." In B. Fleshman (ed.), *Theatrical movement: A bibliographical anthology* (pp. 100–114). Metuchen, N.J.: Scarecrow press.

Middleton, J. (1985). "The dance among the Lugbara of Uganda." In P. Spencer (ed.), *Society and the dance* (pp. 165–182). Cambridge: Cambridge University Press.

Mitchell, J. C. *The Kalela Dance*. Paper No. 17. Manchester: Manchester University Press for the Rhodes-Livingstone Institute.

Moedano, G. (1972). "Los hermanos de la Santa Cuenta: Un culto de crisis de origen Chichimeca." *Religion en Mesoamerica: XXII Mesa Redonda, Sociedad Mexicana de Antropologia*.

Montoye, H. J. (1984). "Exercise and osteoporosis in exercise and health." In H. M. Eckert & H. J. Montoye (ed.), *Exercise and health: American Academy of Physical Education Papers*, No. 17 (pp. 19–75). Champaign, Ill.: Human Kinetics Publishers.

Mooney, J. (1965). *The Ghost-dance religion and the Sioux outbreak of 1890* (ed. by Anthony F. C. Wallace, orig. 1896). Chicago: University of Chicago Press.

Morgan, W. P. (1984). "Physical activity and mental health." In H. M. Eckert & H. J. Montoye (eds.), *Exercise and health: American Academy of Physical Education Papers* No. 17 (pp. 132–145). Champaign, Ill.: Human Kinetics Publishers.

Morgan, W. P. (1985). "Affective beneficence of vigorous physical activity." *Medicine and Science in Sports and Exercise*, 17 (1): 94–100.

Munroe, R. L. (1955). *Schools of psychoanalytic thought: An exposition, critique and attempt at integration*. New York: Holt, Rinehart, and Winston.

Nigerian Government. (1930a). *Aba Commission of Enquiry: Minutes of Evidence*.

———. (1930b). *Report of the commission of inquiry appointed to inquire into the disturbances in the Calabar and Owerri Provinces*, December 1929. Sessional Paper of the Nigerian Legislative Council, No. 28.

Njaka, M. E. N. (1974). *Igbo political culture*. Evanston: Northwestern University Press.

Novack, C. (1984). "Ethnography and history: A case study of dance improvisers." Paper presented at the Dance History Scholars Conference.

Nwabara, S. N. (1965). *Igo land: A study in British penetration and the problem of administration, 1860–1930*. Unpublished doctoral dissertation, Michigan State University.

Nwoga, D. I. (1971). "The concept and practice of satire among the Igbo." *The Conch*, 3 (2): 30–45.

Okonkwo, J. I. (1971). "Adam and Eve: Igbo marriage in the Nigerian novel." *The Conch*, 3 (2): 137–151.

"Onwuteaka, J. D. (1965). "The Aba riot and its relation to the system of indirect rule." *Nigerian Journal of Economic and Social Studies*, November.

Ottenberg, P., and Ottenberg, S. (1964). "Ibo education and social change." In H. N. Weiler (ed.), *Education and politics in Nigeria* (pp. 25–56). Freigburg im Breisgau: Verlag Rombach and Co.

Overby, L. (1986). *A comparison of novice and experienced dancers' imagery ability with respect to their performance on two body awareness tasks*. Unpublished doctoral dissertation, University of Maryland.

Paffenbarger, R., Jr., Hyde, R. T., Wing, A. L., & Hsien, C. (1986). "Physical activity, all-cause morality, and longevity of college alumni." *New England Journal of Medicine*, 314 (10): 605–613.

Panov, V. (1978). *To dance*. New York: Alfred Knopf.

Parks, G. (1986). "New lease on Lar." *Dancemagazine*, 60 (11): 54–56.

Peiss, K. (1986). *Cheap amusements: American working women and leisure in turn-of-the-century New York*. Philadelphia: Temple University Press.

Perham, M. (1937). *Native administration in Nigeria*. London: Oxford University Press.

Pierpont, M. (1984). "At the edge of education—Naropa." *Dancemagazine*, 58 (77): 68–70.

Pollock, M. L., Wilmore, J. H., & Fox III, S. M. (1984). *Exercise in health and disease: Evaluation and prescription for prevention and rehabilitation*. Philadelphia: W. B. Saunders.

Predock-Linnell, J. (nd). *Anxiety and depression in dance: A phenomenological study*. Unpublished paper.

Ranger, T. O. (1975). *Dance and society in Eastern Africa, 1890–1970: The Beni Ngoma.* Berkeley: University of California Press.

Raymond, J. (1979). *Transsexual empire.* Boston: Beacon Press.

Reagan, R. (1983). "Why I quit the ballet." *Newsweek,* February 14, p. 11.

Rockwell, I. (Nadel) (1984). "On stage." *Naropa Magazine,* February, pp. 37–38.

Rockwell, I. (Nadel) (1988). "Dance: The creative process from a contemplative point of view." In L. Y. Overby and J. H. Humphrey (eds.), *Dance: Current selected research.* Vol. I.

Rigby, P. (1966). "Dual symbolic classification among the Gogo of Central Tanzania." *Africa,* 36 (1): 1–17.

Rouget, G. (1985). *Music and trance: A theory of the relations between music and possession* (trans. & rev. by B. Biebuyck). Chicago: University of Chicago Press.

Rovner, S. (1986). "Depression and grief: A biological link." *Washington Post Health,* June 11, p. 6.

Russel, J. F. (1979). "Tarantism." *Medical History,* 23 (4): 404–425.

Sachs, M. & Buffone, G. W. (eds). (1984). *Running as therapy: An integrated approach.* Lincoln: University of Nebraska Press.

Safier, B. (1953). "A psychological orientation to dance and pantomime." *Samiksa,* 7: 236–259.

Sandel, S. L. (1979). "Sexual issues in movement therapy with geriatric patients." *American Journal of Dance Therapy,* 3 (4): 4–14.

Sandel, S. L. (1980). "Countertransference stress in the treatment of schizophrenic patients." *American Journal of Dance Therapy,* 3 (2): 20–32.

Sangree, W. (1969). "Going home to mother: Traditional marriage among the Irigwe, Benue-Plateau State, Nigeria." *American Anthropologist,* 71: 1046–1057.

Schechner, R. (1973). "Drama, script, theatre, and performance." *Drama Review,* 17 (3): 5–36.

Scheff, T. J. (1977). "The distancing of emotion in ritual with CA comment." *Current Anthropology,* 18 (3): 483–505.

Schmais, C. (1985). "Healing processes in group dance therapy." *American Journal of Dance Therapy,* 8: 17–36.

Schneider, M. (1948). *La danza de espadas y la tarentela. Ensayo musicologico, etnografico y arqueologico sobre los ritos medicinales.* Barcelona: Instituto Español de Musicologia.

Schoenfeld, L. (1986). "Dance does it." *Dancemagazine,* 55 (5): 131.

Selye, H. (1974). *Stress without distress.* Philadelphia: J. B. Lippincott.

Selye, H. (1976). *The stress of life*. New York: McGraw Hill.

Selyen, H. (ed.) (1980). *Selye's guide to stress research* Vol. 1. New York: Van Nostrand Reinhold.

Serlin, I. A. (1977). "Portrait of Karen: A gestalt-phenomenological approach to movement therapy." *Journal of Contemporary Psychotherapy,* 8 (2): 145–153.

_____. (1985). *Kinesthetic imagining: A phenomenological study.* Doctoral dissertation, University of Dallas.

Shell, C. G. (ed.). (1986). *The dancer as athlete* (1984 Olympic Scientific Congress Proceedings, Vol. 80). Champaign, Ill.: Human Kinetics Publishers.

Shorter, E. (1982). *A history of women's bodies*. New York: Basic Books.

Siegel, E. V. (1984). *Movement therapy: The mirror of ourselves: A psychoanalytic approach*. New York: Human Sciences Press.

Siegel, M. (1977). *Watching the dance go by*. Boston: Houghton Mifflin.

Silver, J. A. (1981). *Therapeutic aspects of folk dance: Self concept, body concept, ethnic distancing and social distancing*. Doctoral dissertation. University of Toronto.

Smith, E. L. and Serfass, R. (eds.). (1981). *Exercise and aging: The scientific bases*. Hillside, N.J.: Enslow Publishers.

Solway, D. (1986). "In a dancer's world, the inexorable foe is time." *New York Times*, June 8, p. C1, 8.

Sommer, S. R. (1983). "Night in the slammer." *Village Voice*, January 18, pp. 29–31, 106.

Spencer, P. (1985). "Dance as antithesis in the Samburu discourse." In P. Spencer (ed.), *Society and the dance* (pp. 140–164). Cambridge: Cambridge University Press.

Stewart, O. C. (1980). "The Ghost Dance." In W. R. Wood and M. Liberty (eds.), *Anthropology on the great plains* (pp. 179–187). Lincoln: University of Nebraska Press.

Stone, M. (1975). *At the sign of midnight: The Concheros dance cult of Mexico*. Tucson: University of Arizona Press.

Stoop, N. M. (1984). "The Canadian cosmopolitan Montreal's Brian Macdonald." *Dancemagazine*, 58 (4): 62–65.

Tamuno, T. N. (1966). "Before British police in Nigeria." *Nigeria Magazine*, 89: 102–126.

Temin, C. (1982). "The master builder." *Ballet News*, 3 (11): 16–18, 20, 41.

Ten Raa, E. (1969). "The moon as a symbol of life and fertility in Sandawe thought." *Africa*, 39: 24–53.

Thornton, R. (1981). "Demographic antecedents of a revitalization movement, population change, population size, and the 1890 Ghost Dance." *American Sociological Review,* 46 (1): 88–96.

Toffler, A. (1970). *Future shock.* New York: Random House.

Turner, V. (1974). *Dramas, fields, and metaphor: Symbolic action in human society.* Ithaca: Cornell University Press.

Uchendu, V. C. (1965). *The Igbo of Southeast Nigeria.* New York: Holt, Rinehart and Winston.

Umunna, I. (1968). "Igbo names and the concept of death." *African Scholar,* 1 (1): 28.

Van Allen, J. (1972). "'Sitting on a man': Colonialism and the lost political institutions of Igbo women." *Canadian Journal of African Studies,* 6 (2): 165–181.

Vincent, L. M. (1979). *Competing with the sylph: Dancer and the pursuit of the ideal body form.* New York: Andrews and McMeel.

Vogel, M. (1986). "Fit for work: Do on-the-job wellness programs really pay off?" *Washington Post Health,* July 23, pp. 10–13.

Washington Post. (1983). "Stats." April 26, p. B7.

Weisbrod, J. (1974). "Body movement therapy and the visually-impaired person." In K. C. Mason (ed.), *Dance therapy: Focus on Dance VII* (pp. 49–52). Washington, D.C.: American Association for Health, Physical Education and Recreation.

Weston, E. (1982). *A Report: Conference on career transition for dancers.* June 8. New York. Hollywood, Calif.: Actors' Equity Association.

Williams, D. (1968). "The dance of the Bedu moon." *African Arts,* 2 (1): 18–21.

Williams, M. D. (1974). *Community in a black Pentecostal church: An anthropological study.* Pittsburgh: University of Pittsburgh Press.

Wilson, M. (1954). "Nyakyusa ritual and symbolism." *American Anthropologist,* 56: 228–241.

Wolpe, J. (1958). *Psychotherapy by reciprocal inhibition.* Stanford: Stanford University Press.

Wright, S. (1985). *Dancer's guide to injuries of the lower extremity: Diagnosis, treatment and care.* New York: Cornwall Books.

Index